The Utility of Herbicide Exposure Assessment in Epidemiologic Studies of Vietnam Veterans

Committee on Making Best Use of the Agent Orange Exposure
Reconstruction Model

Board on Military and Veterans Health

INSTITUTE OF MEDICINE
OF THE NATIONAL ACADEMIES

THE NATIONAL ACADEMIES PRESS
Washington, D.C.
www.nap.edu

THE NATIONAL ACADEMIES PRESS 500 Fifth Street, N.W. Washington, DC 20001

NOTICE: The project that is the subject of this report was approved by the Governing Board of the National Research Council, whose members are drawn from the councils of the National Academy of Sciences, the National Academy of Engineering, and the Institute of Medicine. The members of the committee responsible for the report were chosen for their special competences and with regard for appropriate balance.

This study was supported by Contract No. V101(93)P-2136 (Task Order #7) between the National Academy of Sciences and the Department of Veterans Affairs. Any opinions, findings, conclusions, or recommendations expressed in this publication are those of the author(s) and do not necessarily reflect the view of the organizations or agencies that provided support for this project.

International Standard Book Number-13: 978-0-309-11449-3
International Standard Book Number-10: 0-309-11449-7

Additional copies of this report are available from the National Academies Press, 500 Fifth Street, N.W., Lockbox 285, Washington, DC 20055; (800) 624-6242 or (202) 334-3313 (in the Washington metropolitan area); Internet, http://www.nap.edu.

For more information about the Institute of Medicine, visit the IOM home page at: **www.iom.edu**.

Copyright 2008 by the National Academy of Sciences. All rights reserved.

Printed in the United States of America.

The serpent has been a symbol of long life, healing, and knowledge among almost all cultures and religions since the beginning of recorded history. The serpent adopted as a logotype by the Institute of Medicine is a relief carving from ancient Greece, now held by the Staatliche Museen in Berlin.

Suggested citation: IOM (Institute of Medicine). 2008. *The utility of proximity-based herbicide exposure assessment in epidemiologic studies in Vietnam veterans.* Washington, DC: The National Academies Press.

*"Knowing is not enough; we must apply.
Willing is not enough; we must do."*
—Goethe

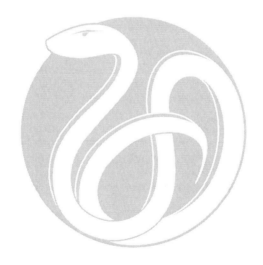

INSTITUTE OF MEDICINE
OF THE NATIONAL ACADEMIES

Advising the Nation. Improving Health.

THE NATIONAL ACADEMIES
Advisers to the Nation on Science, Engineering, and Medicine

The **National Academy of Sciences** is a private, nonprofit, self-perpetuating society of distinguished scholars engaged in scientific and engineering research, dedicated to the furtherance of science and technology and to their use for the general welfare. Upon the authority of the charter granted to it by the Congress in 1863, the Academy has a mandate that requires it to advise the federal government on scientific and technical matters. Dr. Ralph J. Cicerone is president of the National Academy of Sciences.

The **National Academy of Engineering** was established in 1964, under the charter of the National Academy of Sciences, as a parallel organization of outstanding engineers. It is autonomous in its administration and in the selection of its members, sharing with the National Academy of Sciences the responsibility for advising the federal government. The National Academy of Engineering also sponsors engineering programs aimed at meeting national needs, encourages education and research, and recognizes the superior achievements of engineers. Dr. Charles M. Vest is president of the National Academy of Engineering.

The **Institute of Medicine** was established in 1970 by the National Academy of Sciences to secure the services of eminent members of appropriate professions in the examination of policy matters pertaining to the health of the public. The Institute acts under the responsibility given to the National Academy of Sciences by its congressional charter to be an adviser to the federal government and, upon its own initiative, to identify issues of medical care, research, and education. Dr. Harvey V. Fineberg is president of the Institute of Medicine.

The **National Research Council** was organized by the National Academy of Sciences in 1916 to associate the broad community of science and technology with the Academy's purposes of furthering knowledge and advising the federal government. Functioning in accordance with general policies determined by the Academy, the Council has become the principal operating agency of both the National Academy of Sciences and the National Academy of Engineering in providing services to the government, the public, and the scientific and engineering communities. The Council is administered jointly by both Academies and the Institute of Medicine. Dr. Ralph J. Cicerone and Dr. Charles M. Vest are chair and vice chair, respectively, of the National Research Council.

www.national-academies.org

COMMITTEE ON MAKING BEST USE OF THE AGENT ORANGE EXPOSURE RECONSTRUCTION MODEL

DAVID A. SAVITZ (*Chair*), Charles W. Bluhdorn Professor of Community and Preventive Medicine, Director, Epidemiology, Biostatistics, and Disease Prevention Institute, Mount Sinai School of Medicine
MEHRAN ALAEE, Research Scientist, Aquatic Ecosystem Protection Research Division, Environment Canada
FRANCESCA DOMINICI, Professor, Department of Biostatistics, Johns Hopkins Bloomberg School of Public Health
GURUMURTHY RAMACHANDRAN, Professor, Division of Environmental Health Sciences, University of Minnesota
WILLIAM G. SEIBERT, Chief, Archival Operations Branch, Archival Programs Division, National Personnel Records Center, St. Louis, Missouri
LESLIE STAYNER, Professor and Director, Division of Epidemiology and Biostatistics, School of Public Health, University of Illinois at Chicago
LANCE A. WALLER, Professor, Department of Biostatistics, Rollins School of Public Health, Emory University
MARY H. WARD, Investigator, Occupational and Environmental Epidemiology Branch, Division of Cancer Epidemiology and Genetics, National Cancer Institute, National Institutes of Health, Department of Health and Human Services
THOMAS F. WEBSTER, Associate Professor, Department of Environmental Health, Boston University School of Public Health
SUSAN WOSKIE, Professor, Department of Work Environment, University of Massachusetts Lowell

Project Staff

LOIS JOELLENBECK, Senior Program Officer
JANE S. DURCH, Senior Program Officer
JON Q. SANDERS, Program Associate
FREDERICK ERDTMANN, Director, Board on Military and Veterans Health
PAMELA RAMEY McCRAY, Administrative Assistant
ANDREA COHEN, Financial Associate

Reviewers

This report has been reviewed in draft form by individuals chosen for their diverse perspectives and technical expertise, in accordance with procedures approved by the National Research Council's (NRC's) Report Review Committee. The purpose of this independent review is to provide candid and critical comments that will assist the institution in making its published report as sound as possible and to ensure that the report meets institutional standards for objectivity, evidence, and responsiveness to the study charge. The review comments and draft manuscript remain confidential to protect the integrity of the deliberative process. We wish to thank the following individuals for their review of this report:

John C. Bailar III, University of Chicago
Jan Beyea, Consulting in the Public Interest
Norman Breslow, University of Washington
S. Katherine Hammond, School of Public Health, University of California, Berkeley
Ilene Kesselman, Lockheed Martin Corporation
Eric Reiner, Ontario Ministry of the Environment
Peggy Reynolds, Northern California Cancer Center
John E. Vena, Arnold School of Public Health, University of South Carolina
Michael Yost, School of Public Health and Community Medicine, University of Washington

Although the reviewers listed above have provided many constructive comments and suggestions, they were not asked to endorse the conclusions or recommendations, nor did they see the final draft of the report before its release. The review of this report was overseen by **Dan G. Blazer,** Duke University Medical Center, and **Chris G. Whipple,** ENVIRON. Appointed by the NRC and Institute of Medicine, they were responsible for making certain that an independent examination of this report was carried out in accordance with institutional procedures and that all review comments were carefully considered. Responsibility for the final content of this report rests entirely with the authoring committee and the institution.

Preface

Committee reports ultimately reflect the collective wisdom of the individuals who served. I believe that our committee provided the full complement of essential technical skills, gave conscientious effort, and ultimately achieved the needed blend of individual voices to respond in consensus to a complex question. Lois Joellenbeck and Jane Durch kept us focused and ensured progress while carefully avoiding influencing the nature of our conclusions, and they deserve much praise for their skillful leadership.

Despite more than 30 years of efforts to evaluate whether herbicide spraying affected the health of veterans who served in Vietnam, controversy continues and will likely never be put to rest. With unresolved scientific issues regarding the health effects of the chemicals of concern, most notably the contaminant TCDD (2,3,7,8-tetrachlorodibenzo-p-dioxin), and varying judgments regarding the prevalence and levels of exposure experienced by the troops, the Department of Veterans Affairs (VA) has turned to systematic reviews of the epidemiologic and toxicologic evidence by Institute of Medicine committees as a way to synthesize the evidence and guide decisions on compensation. A growing list of conditions has been deemed to be deserving of compensation, with the presumption that those who served in Vietnam were potentially exposed. Controversy is perhaps inevitable given VA's need to face the challenge of how to balance scientific evidence with the obligation to care for the veterans.

Our committee contended with just one specific piece of this very complex array of issues—the best use of a model to characterize exposure to the troops based on their proximity to herbicide spraying in Vietnam.

However, even with a seemingly focused question, it is not possible (or desirable) to ignore the whole array of issues concerning veterans' health. We faced a number of such issues, including what it would mean if the more refined research using this model provided results that did not support compensation decisions already made, the value of using this model to study veterans' health in terms of both the scientific contributions to be made and responsiveness to public concerns, and, even more broadly, the potential for improved but still imperfect research to do more good than harm in this charged context.

We had the opportunity to hear from those who developed the model and defended its merits and others who were highly critical of the model's quality and its potential for making contributions to research. We considered the feasibility of implementing the model in light of the available records on troop locations and movement. We considered the potential contributions of this research tool to learning fundamental information about human health effects of exposure to the herbicides and contaminants of concern, especially TCDD.

We ultimately came to agree that, despite unavoidable and substantial uncertainty about the herbicide exposure of Vietnam veterans, there is value in direct studies of the health of these veterans largely because it is their health that is the issue at hand. The incremental improvement in classifying herbicide exposure during service in Vietnam that the model appears to offer, and the application of that information to studies of veterans' health, has value because of its potential to enhance our understanding of the health experience of this population.

No one on the committee viewed the model and its proximity-based approach to exposure assessment as the silver bullet to resolve all the scientific, compensation, or political controversies surrounding the health of Vietnam veterans. In fact, our greatest concern was the potential for misinterpretation of studies that use this model—that they would be over-interpreted as establishing some "bottom line" finding that would trump the cumulative evidence from studies of herbicides' health effects in other populations with higher and better measured exposures. If in fact there were a perfect system for measuring herbicide exposure and health outcomes in those who served in Vietnam, it might provide hope for a true bottom line, but even with future refinements, this model does not hold out that promise. Should our recommendations be followed and a series of studies making use of the model emerge, the evidence they generate will be only one contribution among many relevant approaches to addressing the potential link between herbicide exposure and health among veterans. In fact, we recognize that in allocating resources, investing in research using the exposure assessment model to study veterans' health is but one among an array of strategies for reducing scientific uncertainty about the health effects of herbicides used in Vietnam and may or may not be the most promising.

We deliberated carefully and reached a series of conclusions that should help VA decide how to proceed on this issue. With our enumeration of the strengths and limitations of the approach, there is no need to be distracted by those who focus only on its limitations or only on its merits, when both perspectives are valid to varying degrees. If some people advocate for the use of this model as the definitive solution to all the underlying controversy and problems in this field, then the balanced review we provide should counter their arguments. Similarly, the committee's review also counters those who would dismiss the approach out of hand due to questions regarding the model's assumptions.

We have tried to provide comprehensive and objective information about what is ultimately a policy decision: whether to invest the resources to improve, evaluate, and apply the exposure assessment model in health studies. In light of the questions that remain concerning herbicide exposure and health among Vietnam veterans and the array of evidence that has thus far been brought to bear on that issue, we believe that the application of this model and its potential refinements offers a constructive approach to extending knowledge about the effects of herbicides on the health of these veterans and merits the initial steps recommended in our report.

David Savitz
Chair

Acknowledgments

Many individuals assisted the committee in its work by providing useful data and presenting information at the committee's public meetings. We thank the following people for participating in the committee's public meetings: Mark Brown and Han Kang, Department of Veterans Affairs; Jeanne Mager Stellman, SUNY Downstate Medical Center (formerly at Columbia University); Steven Stellman, Columbia University; Richard Boylan, National Archives and Records Administration; David Garabrant, University of Michigan School of Public Health; John Giesy, University of Saskatchewan; Michael Ginevan, M.E. Ginevan and Associates; Donald Hakenson, U.S. Army and Joint Services Records Research Center; Shannon Middleton, American Legion; John Ross, Infoscientific.com, Inc.; Thomas Sinks, Centers for Disease Control and Prevention; Marie Haring Sweeney, National Institute for Occupational Safety and Health; David Tollerud, University of Louisville; Richard Weidman, Vietnam Veterans of America; and Alvin Young, *Environmental Science and Pollution Research* (editor). The committee also wishes to thank the following individuals who made information available to the committee and study staff: Drue Barrett, Centers for Disease Control and Prevention; Thomas Boivin, Hatfield Consultants; Tim Bullman and Yasmin Cypel, Department of Veterans Affairs; Keith Horsley, Australian Institute of Health and Welfare; and Sang-Wook Yi, Kwandong University, South Korea. In addition, Institute of Medicine (IOM) staff members David Butler, Harriet Crawford, William Page, and Mary Paxton met with the committee and aided the study staff in the collection and analysis of background material.

The committee offers special thanks to Jeanne Mager Stellman and Steven Stellman, who participated in the committee's three public meetings and responded to several requests for supplemental information. Our project officer from the Department of Veterans Affairs, Mark Brown, provided valuable guidance on the scope of the study as the committee began its work. Also at the Department of Veterans Affairs, Han Kang responded to several requests for additional information.

Thanks go as well to other members of the staff of the Institute of Medicine and the National Academies. As a member of the study staff, Jon Sanders ably ensured that logistical and information needs were met. Also supporting the study were Frederick (Rick) Erdtmann, Director, Board on Military and Veterans Health; Andrea Cohen, Financial Associate; Bronwyn Schrecker Jamrok, Manager, IOM Report Review; and Lara Andersen, Senior Editorial Manager. In addition, Robert Pool provided helpful editorial services.

Contents

ACRONYMS AND ABBREVIATIONS		xvii
SUMMARY		1
1	INTRODUCTION AND BACKGROUND	13
	Study Charge and Committee Activities, 14	
	A Brief History, 15	
	Issues in Assessing Herbicide Exposure in Vietnam for Epidemiologic Studies, 21	
	The Committee's Report, 22	
	References, 22	
2	THE HERBICIDE EXPOSURE ASSESSMENT MODEL	25
	The Exposure Opportunity Concept, 26	
	Components of the Herbicide Exposure Assessment Model, 29	
	Unit Location Information, 32	
	References, 33	
3	ASSESSMENT OF THE MODEL AND ITS CAPACITY TO PRODUCE USEFUL EXPOSURE METRICS	35
	An Exposure Assessment Hierarchy for Vietnam Veterans, 36	
	Infrastructure of the Stellman Team's Model, 39	
	Evaluation of the Infrastructure of the Stellman Team's Model, 43	
	The Stellman Team's Exposure Opportunity Metrics, 45	

Evaluation of the Stellman Team's Exposure Opportunity
    Metrics, 46
Potential for Corroboration of Exposure Measures, 53
Testing and Refining the Stellman Team's Model, 57
Conclusions, 59
Research Opportunities, 60
References, 61

4   DATA FOR EPIDEMIOLOGIC STUDIES OF
    VIETNAM VETERANS   65
    Available Troop Location Data, 65
    Obtaining Additional Troop Location Data from Military
        Records, 68
    Sources of Health Outcome Information, 76
    Conclusions, 80
    References, 81

5   RECOMMENDATIONS REGARDING EPIDEMIOLOGIC
    STUDIES USING THE EXPOSURE ASSESSMENT MODEL   84
    Should Studies Be Done Using the Stellman Team's Model?, 84
    Contributions and Pitfalls of Studies Using the Model, 85
    General Considerations for Conducting Studies, 91
    Types of Studies for Consideration, 97
    Potential Study Populations, 99
    Ongoing VA Work to Apply the Exposure Assessment Model, 104
    Contribution to the Ongoing IOM Reviews of the Association
        Between Herbicide Exposure and Health Outcomes, 106
    Conclusions, 106
    Recommendations, 107
    References, 108

APPENDIXES
A   Agendas for Information-Gathering Meetings   113
B   Exposure Measures in Studies of U.S. Vietnam Veterans   119
C   Biographical Sketches of Committee Members   136

Acronyms and Abbreviations

2,4-D	2,4-dichlorophenoxyacetic acid
2,4,5-T	2,4,5-trichlorophenoxyacetic acid
ALS	amyotrophic lateral sclerosis
ATSDR	Agency for Toxic Substances and Disease Registry
BIRLS	Beneficiary Identification and Record Locator Subsystem
CDC	Centers for Disease Control and Prevention
CMS	Centers for Medicare and Medicaid Services
CRUR	Center for Research of Unit Records
CURR	Center for Unit Records Research
DAAR	Daily Air Activities Report
DMF	Death Master File
DoD	U.S. Department of Defense
EOI	exposure opportunity index
EPA	Environmental Protection Agency
ESG	U.S. Army and Joint Services Environmental Support Group
FOIA	Freedom of Information Act

g	gram
GAO	Government Accountability Office (previously General Accounting Office)
GIS	geographic information system
HEA-V	Herbicide Exposure Assessment–Vietnam
IARC	International Agency for Research on Cancer
IOM	Institute of Medicine
JSRRC	U.S. Army and Joint Services Records Research Center
km	kilometer
MACV	U.S. Military Assistance Command, Vietnam
MFUA	Medical Follow-up Agency
NARA	National Archives and Records Administration
NAS	National Academy of Sciences
NCHS	National Center for Health Statistics
NDI	National Death Index
ng	nanogram
NHL	non-Hodgkin's lymphoma
NLM	National Library of Medicine
NPRC	National Personnel Records Center
NRC	National Research Council
NTIS	National Technical Information Service
OMPF	Official Military Personnel File
OPC	Outpatient Clinic File
PCDD	polychlorinated dibenzodioxin
PCDF	polychlorinated dibenzofuran
pg	picogram
P.L.	Public Law
ppm	parts per million
ppt	parts per trillion
PTF	Patient Treatment File
PTSD	posttraumatic stress disorder
ResDAC	Research Data Assistance Center

SNF	skilled nursing facility
SSA DMF	Social Security Administration's Death Master File
TCDD	2,3,7,8-tetrachlorodibenzo-p-dioxin
USMC	U.S. Marine Corps
UTM	Universal Transverse Mercator coordinate system
VA	U.S. Department of Veterans Affairs

Summary

ABSTRACT *In past studies evaluating whether health problems experienced by Vietnam veterans might be linked to wartime use of Agent Orange or other herbicides, a fundamental challenge has been a lack of information about the veterans' level of exposure to these herbicides. To address that problem, researchers developed a model to assess the opportunity for herbicide exposure among these veterans. Using a geographic information system and a computerized database engine, the model makes it possible to link georeferenced data on herbicide spray paths with information about troop locations and calculate two different proximity-based exposure opportunity metrics. This report presents the conclusions and recommendations of an Institute of Medicine committee that was convened to provide guidance to the Department of Veterans Affairs (VA) about the best use of this herbicide exposure assessment model.*

The committee concluded that the model's approach of using an exposure surrogate based on individuals' or military units' proximity in space and time to herbicide spray paths is a reasonable one. It is an important improvement over the cruder yes/no exposure classification based on service in Vietnam that has been used in many past epidemiologic studies of the health of Vietnam veterans. However, the proximity-based exposure metrics inevitably have some unknown amount of misclassification and must be used and interpreted with caution. Sensitivity analyses should be done to determine the effect that the model's assumptions have on the exposure assignments it generates, and other proximity-based approaches with the potential of estimating exposure more accurately should be explored. Moving beyond proximity-based exposure measures would require additional data on herbicide fate and transport, individual behavior, and pharmacokinetics, and some of this information is not likely to be available.

To conduct epidemiologic studies using the exposure assessment model requires data on when and where each veteran served in Vietnam and on the veteran's health outcomes. It is generally possible to obtain useful data on individuals' unit assignments and unit locations, but the processes of gaining permission for access to relevant military records and of collecting data for individuals are likely to be administratively difficult for many researchers as well as time consuming and costly.

Despite the shortcomings of the exposure assessment model in its current form and the inherent limitations in the approach, the committee agreed that the model holds promise for supporting informative epidemiologic studies of herbicides and health among Vietnam veterans and that it should be used to conduct studies. The committee offers criteria that VA should draw on as a basis for developing a request for proposals, and it recommends that VA work with the Department of Defense and the National Archives and Records Administration to facilitate access to and interpretation of military records for use in the studies.

Between 1962 and 1971, several herbicides—most notably the product known as Agent Orange—were used in Vietnam by U.S. forces and their allies for defoliation of forest areas, destruction of crops, and control of vegetation around the perimeters of troop encampments. Since then, many studies have been conducted to examine whether health problems experienced by some Vietnam veterans might be linked to their wartime exposure to any of these herbicides or to a particular contaminant—2,3,7,8-tetrachlorodibenzo-p-dioxin (TCDD)—that was present in some of them.[1]

A fundamental and persisting challenge in these studies has been to determine the amount of herbicide in the environment in Vietnam, identify military personnel who were exposed to the herbicides, distinguish them from personnel who were not exposed, and estimate the herbicide or dioxin dose that exposed individuals received. In an effort to improve exposure assessment for Vietnam veterans, a group of academic researchers has

---

[1]Throughout this report the term "herbicide" encompasses the TCDD contaminant unless specifically stated otherwise.

developed an herbicide exposure assessment model. This report presents the conclusions and recommendations of the Institute of Medicine (IOM) study committee that was convened to provide guidance to the Department of Veterans Affairs (VA) on the use of this model.

The committee found that assignment of exposure based on proximity to herbicide spraying offers the possibility of important improvement in the classification of exposure over most earlier approaches, although there are inherent limitations in the model. Using the model to assess herbicide exposure in epidemiologic studies may permit observation of associations between herbicide exposure and health effects in the Vietnam veteran population that were not identifiable in previous studies. The committee recommends further sensitivity analyses to provide a better understanding of the model's strengths, limitations, and uncertainties and also recommends exploration of opportunities to refine the model's estimation of exposure.

STUDY BACKGROUND

U.S. military personnel were present in Vietnam throughout the 1962–1971 period when herbicides were in use for defoliation and crop destruction. Among the several different herbicides used, Agent Orange and Agent White were the principal defoliants and Agent Blue was widely used for crop destruction.[2] Available data indicate that 95 percent of the herbicide used in Vietnam was applied by fixed-wing aircraft as part of Operation Ranch Hand. Herbicides were also applied by helicopters and with ground-spraying apparatus. Records for Operation Ranch Hand are considered to be relatively more complete than those for other herbicide use.

In 1991, Congress requested that IOM committees periodically review the scientific evidence to assess whether associations may exist between exposure to the herbicides (or the TCDD contaminant) used in Vietnam and health outcomes. Congress originally sought from the IOM reviews an assessment of the increased risk that Vietnam veterans would have for conditions found to be associated with herbicide exposure. None of the review committees have been able to make quantitative assessments, in part, because credible direct or proxy measurements of Vietnam veterans' herbicide exposure have not been available.

The first of the IOM's biennial reviews included a recommendation that this problem be addressed by an attempt to develop an exposure reconstruction model that could be considered valid for use in epidemiologic studies of veterans. VA responded to this recommendation by com-

---

[2]Agent Orange was a combination of 2,4-dichlorophenoxyacetic acid (2,4-D) and 2,4,5-trichlorophenoxyacetic acid (2,4,5-T). Agent White was a combination of 2,4-D and picloram. Agent Blue was cacodylic acid and sodium cacodylate. TCDD was a contaminant of 2,4,5-T.

missioning the IOM to assess the scientific issues that a research proposal would need to address, to oversee the selection of a contractor to conduct the work, to monitor progress during the course of the contract, and to evaluate the product produced by the contractor. The contract for the work was awarded in 1998 to researchers at the Columbia University Mailman School of Public Health (Jeanne Mager Stellman, Ph.D., principal investigator), who produced the proximity-based exposure assessment model that is the focus of this report.

STUDY CHARGE

The Committee on Making Best Use of the Agent Orange Exposure Reconstruction Model was convened in 2007 to advise VA on the best ways to employ the herbicide exposure assessment model in the evaluation of the long-term health effects of veterans' wartime exposure to herbicides. VA requested that the committee consider several factors: the relevant IOM recommendations for evaluating such a model; approaches for evaluating the exposure model using existing data on health outcomes associated with herbicide or dioxin exposure among Vietnam veterans; the availability, quality, and usefulness of existing information on Vietnam veterans, including data on troop locations and health outcomes for diseases commonly associated with herbicide exposure as well as those not currently linked to such exposures; and how such information might be used in epidemiologic studies using the exposure assessment model. The committee was also asked to consider the role of epidemiologic studies of Vietnam veterans conducted using the new model in informing the IOM's biennial evaluation of evidence on the association between herbicide exposure and health outcomes. VA's interests included advice on planning future research using the model, guiding researchers to the potentially most fruitful areas of study, and alerting researchers to the challenges in doing studies using the model.

Despite the name of the committee, it is important to note that the herbicide exposure assessment model that was reviewed is not an *exposure reconstruction* model. To the committee, "exposure reconstruction" suggests the possibility of arriving at a retrospective estimate of the quantity of herbicide that individuals or groups were exposed to, or even the dose they might have received. Instead, the model produces metrics based on proximity to herbicide spraying that are only surrogates for exposure. Furthermore, the committee was not charged with conducting analyses using the exposure assessment model or with conducting an assessment of the scientific evidence on associations between any specific health effects and exposure to herbicides used in Vietnam.

AN EXPOSURE ASSESSMENT HIERARCHY

The committee viewed the Stellman team's exposure assessment model in the context of an exposure assessment hierarchy for herbicide spraying in Vietnam (see Figure 3-1). At the simplest level, "exposure" is defined based on a veteran's presence or absence in Vietnam during the period of herbicide spraying. Measures of exposure at the second level are based on information on the location, timing, and volume of herbicide spraying combined with information on the location in space and time of individuals or military units. At the third level, proximity-based exposure metrics might be refined by the incorporation of more detailed data or models for the fate and transport of herbicides in the environment, such as spray drift models, estimates of the proportion of the sprayed herbicide that reached the ground, or consideration of secondary transport of the herbicides or the TCDD contaminant in the environment. The fourth level of the hierarchy would require data on individual-level interactions with the environment (e.g., dermal exposure to soil, consumption of local food) to better estimate personal exposures and permit examination of differences among units or individuals present at the same places and times. At the fifth and most highly refined level, information on pharmacokinetics would be needed to estimate the doses of a toxic compound that individuals receive.

The Stellman team's model operates primarily at the second level of this hierarchy, relating the location of military units in time and space to the timing, location, and volume of herbicide spraying. Understanding this aspect of the model is necessary in order to accurately evaluate its strengths and weaknesses and to advise future researchers about its appropriate use.

A TOOL FOR HERBICIDE EXPOSURE ASSESSMENT

The Stellman team developed a geographic information system (GIS) and the Herbicide Exposure Assessment–Vietnam (HEA-V), which is a computerized database engine that facilitates the linking of disparate georeferenced data as well as the calculation of two exposure opportunity metrics at the spatial scale of approximately 1 square kilometer.

The "hits" metric is based on an individual's or a unit's presence at a given location within a specified distance from a spray path at the time of a spray mission. Hits are calculated for each cell in the GIS grid that lies within 0.5, 1, 2, or 5 kilometers of a spray path. The other metric is the Exposure Opportunity Index (EOI), which factors in both direct exposure and an estimate of indirect exposure to residual herbicide from spraying that occurred before an individual's or a unit's entry into a location. The EOI calculations incorporate data on the quantity of herbicide sprayed, the distance from the spray path, the time since spraying, and an environmental half-life. Hits and EOIs can be calculated for a specific location or for military units or individual military personnel when their location histories are provided.

CONSIDERATIONS IN ASSESSING HERBICIDE EXPOSURE IN VIETNAM FOR EPIDEMIOLOGIC STUDIES

The committee's assessment was guided by four primary considerations. First, it was essential to be clear about the nature of the exposure assessment model and what it does and does not claim to do. The committee approached the model as a means of generating a quantitative representation of *opportunity* for herbicide exposure, acknowledging that it could not provide sophisticated estimates of individual dose or exposure levels.

Second, the committee gave careful consideration to the information needed to use the model. This included gaining an understanding of the strengths and limitations of data on herbicide spraying, troop locations, and health outcomes. Issues of access to and usability of these data were also important. Although attention in the past has often focused on TCDD, the spraying database includes information on all herbicides for which records were available, and the committee made its assessment from this broader perspective.

Third, the committee considered whether the model "works," that is, whether it locates spraying and troops accurately (opportunity for exposure) and whether doing so is related to actual exposure (through comparisons with other sources of information on exposure, such as blood levels or environmental samples). Because environmental epidemiology often advances through successive approximations of exposure and not necessarily by applying the standard of absolute accuracy, the utility of the model is defined in part by the methods it improves upon.

Fourth, with the nature of the model and its metrics clearly in mind, the committee considered the potential contributions and pitfalls of using it in epidemiologic studies. Of particular interest in these deliberations were the potential to study Vietnam veterans directly, the degree to which exposure classification might be improved if the model were to be used, and the appropriate interpretation of the results of any such studies.

ASSESSMENT OF THE MODEL AND ITS EXPOSURE METRICS

The committee considered it necessary to assess the strengths and weaknesses of the Stellman team's approach to herbicide exposure assessment before commenting on the best use of the model. This initial assessment focused on (1) the basic data inputs on geography and herbicide spraying, (2) the exposure metrics of hits and EOI, and (3) the assumptions regarding the effects of distance from spraying in time and space that are incorporated into the calculation of the EOI.

Infrastructure for Proximity-Based Exposure Measures

The committee concluded that the Stellman team's approach of using an exposure surrogate based on individuals' or military units' proximity in space and time to herbicide spray paths is a reasonable exposure assessment strategy. This approach is an important improvement over the cruder exposure classification based on service in Vietnam that has been used in many past studies of the health of Vietnam veterans.

The databases and GIS were found to provide a useful infrastructure for estimating proximity-based surrogates of exposure to herbicides in Vietnam. However, data on spraying by fixed-wing aircraft are more complete than the data for spraying by ground equipment or helicopters. As a result, the model is currently better suited to examining proximity to fixed-wing spraying. Even so, it is important for the potential contribution of herbicide exposures from helicopter and ground spraying to be taken into consideration in planning and interpreting studies, recognizing that sources of exposure other than from fixed-wing aircraft could introduce misclassification in the rank-order of exposure assignment.

In addition, given the significant uncertainties in the levels of TCDD contamination in the herbicides used in Vietnam, proximity-based exposure models may be better suited to studies of the health effects of herbicides for which the active ingredients were consistent over time, such as 2,4-D and 2,4,5-T, rather than TCDD. Should researchers want to distinguish between proximity to Agent Orange and proximity to Agent White or Agent Blue, for example, it is possible to generate separate exposure opportunity values for each agent using the Stellman team's model.

The committee concluded that the proximity-based exposure metrics of hits and EOI have value in that they move in a favorable direction along the exposure assessment hierarchy described above. However, the methods by which the hits and EOI scores are calculated have the potential for exposure misclassification of unknown magnitude, and so these metrics must be used with caution. Other proximity-based approaches to estimating exposure may be more accurate and should be explored using the existing GIS. Moving beyond proximity-based measures would require additional data on meteorologic conditions, herbicide fate and transport, individual behavior, and pharmacokinetics.

Testing and Refining Herbicide Exposure Assessment

The Committee concluded that factors influencing the environmental fate and transport of the herbicides that were not incorporated into the current version of the Stellman team's model (e.g., width of the spray swath, concentration of contaminants, primary and secondary drift, soil conditions, initial and remaining canopy, and photodegradation) are likely to have affected exposure to herbicides and their contaminants. Incorporating these phenomena into an exposure model could possibly reduce exposure misclassification, but it would require additional data that may or may not be available. Furthermore, the resolution of the Universal Transverse Mercator (UTM) system used in the military records and the approximately 1-square-kilometer resolution of the Stellman team's GIS grid map of Vietnam limits to some extent the benefits of adding fine-scale fate and transport modeling.

The committee emphasizes that, regardless of the exposure model used, sensitivity analyses are necessary to determine the impact of the model's assumptions on the exposure assignments it generates. In addition, the committee concluded that it is not feasible to validate the exposure scores produced by the Stellman team's model—or any other proximity-based model—by comparisons with biomarkers or soil samples because of the passage of time and the unavailability of archived environmental or biological samples.

AVAILABILITY AND ACCESSIBILITY OF DATA ON VETERANS

The Stellman team's herbicide exposure assessment model starts from a data infrastructure that focuses on the timing, location, and content of herbicide spraying in Vietnam and the software tools for calculating exposure metrics. To generate exposure metrics that can be used in epidemiologic studies, this infrastructure must be supplemented with data on when and where military personnel served in Vietnam and on their health outcomes.

Working with the Joint Services Records Research Center at the Department of Defense (DoD) and with records held by the National Archives and Records Administration (NARA), the Stellman team has assembled location data for many of the military units that moved infrequently during the time they served in Vietnam (i.e., stable units) as well as for some combat units, which moved frequently. Conducting a person-based study requires the further step of identifying the individuals who served in these units and gaining access to their military records. However, access to this information is constrained by privacy laws and is especially challenging for researchers who are not affiliated with DoD or VA.

The committee concluded that it is generally possible to obtain useful data on individuals' unit assignments and unit locations. Locations for most stationary units have already been catalogued, and it appears feasible to gather adequate location information for mobile troops. However, the processes of gaining permission for access to relevant military records and of collecting data for individuals are likely to be administratively difficult for many researchers, as well as time consuming and costly. Assistance from experts in the location and interpretation of Vietnam-era military records is likely to be essential for the effective collection of data from these sources.

Epidemiologic studies will also require assembling mortality or morbidity data for Vietnam veterans. With appropriate identifying information, mortality data for Vietnam veterans are readily and reliably available through the National Death Index and the Social Security Administration's Death Master File. Mortality data can also be obtained from VA's Beneficiary Identification and Record Locator Subsystem (BIRLS), but access to this database is more limited.

Obtaining morbidity data presents greater challenges. VA has several databases that could contribute information about the health status of some veterans, but only about 20 percent of Vietnam veterans are receiving care from the VA, and access to VA data is typically restricted to VA researchers. However, as more Vietnam veterans reach age 65 and become eligible for Medicare, it will be possible to use Medicare records to conduct morbidity studies. Researchers could also explore other resources such as state cancer registries and hospital discharge datasets.

The committee notes that the Air Force Ranch Hand personnel and Army Chemical Corps personnel are two groups of veterans that are not suitable study populations when the Stellman team's model is to be used, even though their exposures to herbicides are likely to be among the highest of all veterans. Most of their herbicide exposures were a direct result of duties that required handling or applying herbicides. By contrast, the model is designed to assess the exposure opportunity that would result from unintended proximity to herbicide spraying.

EPIDEMIOLOGIC STUDIES USING THE HERBICIDE EXPOSURE ASSESSMENT MODEL

Despite recognizing shortcomings in the exposure assessment model in its current form and inherent limitations in the proximity-based approach, the committee concluded that the assessment model holds promise for contributing to informative epidemiologic studies of herbicides and health among Vietnam veterans and that it should be used to conduct such studies.

Two key considerations led to this conclusion. First, the exposure assessment model is applicable to the population of ultimate interest, namely Vietnam veterans. No other group has the confluence of exposures and exposure circumstances experienced by the Vietnam veterans, so given an adequate model, there is inherent value in asking the question in this group.

Second, many previous studies of this population have been severely limited with respect to exposure assessment. A more accurate, if still imperfect, method should increase the specificity of exposure classification and may permit observation of associations between herbicide exposure and health effects in the Vietnam veteran population that were not identifiable in previous studies.

The committee also concluded that the ongoing work by VA investigators is constructive in characterizing the logistical challenges and magnitude of effort needed to apply the Stellman team's herbicide exposure assessment model. However, the committee views this work as too limited and insufficiently accessible to the broader research community to constitute, in isolation, the best use of the model.

Two types of study design were judged to be the most promising for application of the model. One approach is a cohort study that would start from military units and identify individual veterans who served in those units. Units might be selectively sampled based on their exposure potential. The other approach suggested by the committee is to build on large cohorts already assembled and pursue nested case-control studies of outcomes of interest within those cohorts. Either approach would require assembling location histories for individual study subjects.

Efforts to validate the model solely by examining existing data on health outcomes associated with herbicide exposure are of limited value. If positive, such studies would add support to the model's potential value, but if negative, the model's value is not disproved because the levels of exposure may be lower than would cause adverse health effects or the study's power may be insufficient to address the question adequately.

Studies of veterans based on the exposure assessment model should include analyses to assess how sensitive an estimated association between the exposure opportunity metric and specific health outcomes is to different parameters and sources of uncertainty in the exposure assessment measure. Sensitivity analyses that summarize the variability in the model's exposure metrics under different assumptions underlying the exposure opportunity model will provide ranges and distributions of exposure opportunity metrics (hits or EOI) that may be included in statistical estimates, such as rate ratios and logistic regression parameters. In this way, researchers can offer a range or distribution of the estimated risks associated with the exposure and so illuminate the underlying uncertainty in the assumptions of the model.

In order for other researchers to benefit from such analyses as well as any refinements or extensions of the model, the committee encourages those who conduct studies applying the exposure assessment model not only to address meaningful epidemiologic questions but also to follow the example set by the Stellman team in contributing publicly accessible building blocks for reanalyses and refinements by others. Work that investigators—including VA researchers—carry out to determine unit locations and calculations used to arrive at exposure indices should be documented and made available, ideally through the Internet, to enable others to repeat the analyses. Any extension or refinement of the model and associated sensitivity analyses should also be documented so that others can evaluate and build upon the work.

RECOMMENDATIONS

The committee's conclusions from its consideration of the Stellman team's herbicide exposure assessment model led it to make the following recommendations:

1. **VA should sponsor epidemiologic studies of Vietnam veterans that take into account the criteria below regarding the appropriate characteristics of informative research on herbicide exposure and health outcomes in this population. VA should draw on the criteria as the basis for developing a request for proposals.**

    Specifically, to make the best use of the exposure assessment model, epidemiologic studies of Vietnam veterans should have the following characteristics:

    a. The study population should be broadly representative of Vietnam veterans, with care taken to include sufficient numbers of study participants with relatively higher exposure.
    b. A broad range of health outcomes should be considered, not just those that are suspected of being related to herbicide exposure. Where feasible, morbidity should be studied in addition to mortality.
    c. The health data should be as complete and up-to-date as possible.
    d. The study should have sufficient statistical power to address the range of health outcomes of concern.
    e. To isolate the effects of herbicide exposure, potential confounding factors need to be carefully addressed in the study design or the analytic approach.

f. Analyses should be conducted to evaluate how sensitive the estimated associations between exposure opportunity and health outcomes are to the uncertainty in the exposure opportunity metrics and to varying approaches to estimating herbicide exposure, possibly including alternative approaches to exposure assignment as discussed in Chapter 3.
g. Opportunities to conduct research using the exposure assessment model should be open to investigators beyond the VA system to allow for the benefits of engaging the broader research community and to enhance public acceptance and credibility.

2. In support of the recommended epidemiologic studies, VA should work with DoD and NARA to

- facilitate health research uses of military records that are subject to access barriers arising from privacy laws, and
- arrange for assistance from DoD and NARA staff with appropriate expertise to aid researchers in the location and interpretation of military records for health research uses.

RESEARCH OPPORTUNITIES

From its review of the Stellman team's model, the committee also identified two areas where it urges further investigation.

First, efforts should be made to improve and refine the Stellman team's model by exploring alternative formulations of the proximity-based exposure metrics and by incorporating alternative or additional model parameters that account for more aspects of herbicide fate and transport in the environment. Further development of the model will require an assessment of the additional data needed and the availability of these data.

Second, the sensitivity of the Stellman team's model's results to changes in parameter values should be assessed systematically. The committee specifically urges attention to the effects of potential inaccuracies in the data on the location of herbicide application or troop presence. It is also important to investigate, especially with any attempt to add refinements to the existing model, the effect of assumptions on factors such as spray swath, the concentration of the TCDD contamination, primary and secondary drift, soil conditions, initial and remaining canopy, and photodegradation of sprayed herbicide. Although the committee concluded, based on the information it reviewed, that direct validation of the accuracy of exposure assignment is not feasible, it encourages efforts to quantify the degree of accuracy and incorporate those estimates into the sensitivity analysis.

1

Introduction and Background

Between 1962 and 1971, several herbicides—most notably the product known as Agent Orange—were used in Vietnam by U.S. forces and their allies for defoliation of forest areas, destruction of crops, and control of vegetation around the perimeters of troop encampments. Since then many studies have been conducted to examine whether health problems experienced by some Vietnam veterans might be linked to wartime exposure to any of these herbicides or to a contaminant (i.e., 2,3,7,8-tetrachlorodibenzo-*p*-dioxin [TCDD]) that was in some of them.[1]

A fundamental and persisting challenge in these studies has been to determine the amount of herbicide in the wartime environment, identify the military personnel who were exposed to herbicides, distinguish them from personnel who were not exposed, and estimate the herbicide or TCDD dose that exposed individuals received. In response to a recommendation in the Institute of Medicine (IOM) report *Veterans and Agent Orange: Health Effects of Herbicides Used in Vietnam* (IOM, 1994) that an effort to develop models to reconstruct herbicide exposure be undertaken, the Department of Veterans Affairs (VA) funded and the IOM (1997, 2003a,b) oversaw work by researchers at Columbia University to produce an herbicide exposure assessment model (Stellman and Stellman, 2003, 2004; Stellman et al., 2003a,b).

VA subsequently sought advice from IOM on the use of the exposure assessment model in epidemiologic studies to evaluate the long-term health

---

[1] Throughout this report the term "herbicide" encompasses the TCDD contaminant unless specifically stated otherwise.

effects of wartime exposure to herbicides. This report presents the conclusions and recommendations of the IOM study committee convened to provide this guidance to VA.

STUDY CHARGE AND COMMITTEE ACTIVITIES

The IOM study requested by VA has the following Statement of Task:

> A committee will be convened to provide the U.S. Department of Veterans Affairs with advice and suggestions on the best ways to employ the "Agent Orange" exposure assessment model developed by Columbia University researchers in the evaluation of the long-term health effects of wartime exposure to herbicides. VA has requested that the committee include the following in their considerations:
>
> - The relevant recommendations for evaluating the model contained in the 1994 report *Veterans and Agent Orange*.
> - Approaches to evaluating the exposure model using existing data on health outcomes associated with herbicide or dioxin exposure among Vietnam veterans.
> - The availability, quality, and usefulness of existing information on Vietnam veterans, including troop locations and health outcome data regarding diseases commonly associated with herbicide exposure (soft tissue sarcoma, non-Hodgkin's lymphoma, Hodgkin's disease, or lung and laryngeal cancer, for example) as well as those not currently linked to such exposures (e.g., testicular, colon, or skin cancer).
> - How such information might be used in studies that would become the basis of further epidemiological research using the exposure reconstruction model.
> - The role of epidemiologic studies of Vietnam veterans using the new model in informing the evaluation of the association between herbicide exposure and health outcomes performed in the Veterans and Agent Orange–series reports.
>
> The committee will prepare a report describing its work and offering findings and recommendations.

The study committee was selected to include members with expertise in environmental and occupational epidemiology, exposure assessment, environmental health, environmental chemistry, biostatistics, and access to archived military records.

The committee met in person four times from March 2007 through August 2007. During these meetings, the committee reviewed and discussed the existing research literature on the topics central to its charge and received information from oral presentations made by the researchers who developed the exposure assessment model, by researchers studying dioxin and herbicide contamination in the United States and Vietnam, and by representatives from VA, the Centers for Disease Control and Prevention (CDC), and veterans service organizations. (See Appendix A for the agendas of the information-gathering meetings.) In addition, the committee met via a conference call to complete its deliberations.

Despite the name of the committee, it is important to note that the herbicide exposure assessment model that was reviewed is not an *exposure reconstruction* model. To the committee, "exposure reconstruction" suggests the possibility of arriving at a retrospective estimate of the quantity of herbicide that individuals or groups were exposed to, or even the dose they might have received. Instead, the model produces metrics based on proximity to herbicide spraying that are only surrogates for exposure. Furthermore, the committee was not charged with conducting analyses using the exposure assessment model or with conducting an assessment of the scientific evidence on associations between any specific health effects and exposure to herbicides used in Vietnam.

A BRIEF HISTORY

This chapter provides readers with brief background information on the size of the population of U.S. military personnel who served in Vietnam, the herbicides used there, the response to concerns about potential health effects of exposure to these herbicides, and findings from other IOM studies on associations between health effects and herbicide exposure.

U.S. Military Personnel in Vietnam

U.S. military troops were present in Vietnam from the 1950s until 1973 (IOM, 1994). Herbicides were in use from 1962 through 1971, making persons who served during that period the population of interest for epidemiologic studies. Table 1-1 shows (fiscal) year-end troop levels in Vietnam for 1960–1973, based on data currently available from the Department of Defense (DoD, 2007). Although data on the numbers of troops present in Vietnam have been available (if not always entirely consistent) since the end of the war, identifying specific individuals who served there has been more challenging. A computerized roster of approximately 3 million military personnel who are thought to have served in Vietnam was not compiled by DoD and VA until the mid-1990s (Kang, 2007). This roster is discussed further in Chapter 5.

Summary data on the length of time individuals served in Vietnam do not appear to have been compiled. The U.S. Army had an individual rotation policy with 1-year tours in South Vietnam (The U.S. Army in Vietnam, 2005; DePue, 2006). The Marine Corps adopted an individual rotation

TABLE 1-1 U.S. Troop Levels in Vietnam, by Branch of Service, 1960–1973[a]

Year	Total	Army	Navy	Marine Corps	Air Force[b]
1960	794	558	98	21	117
1961	959	701	105	20	133
1962	8,464	6,747	338	720	659
1963	15,575	10,878	606	233	3,858
1964	17,033	10,892	574	761	4,806
1965	124,363	75,025	1,691	37,179	10,468
1966	305,183	192,975	9,109	58,624	44,475
1967	437,103	294,962	12,784	74,660	54,697
1968	537,377	354,212	38,388	83,873	60,904
1969	510,054	345,423	33,708	71,239	59,684
1970	390,278	294,088	19,497	29,962	46,731
1971	212,925	167,304	10,308	459	34,854
1972	35,292	21,212	1,997	1,290	10,793
1973	265	31	3	167	64

[a]Status on September 30 of each year. The data include only land-based personnel.
[b]These data are based on the permanent duty location of individuals and thus differ from Air Force deployment data by command, which reflect the headquarters location of organizational units.
SOURCE: DoD, 2007.

policy in 1965, and Marines served a 12- or 13-month tour in Vietnam (USMC, 1985). The number of service members who served multiple tours is not known.

Herbicide Use in Vietnam

Use of herbicides for defoliation and crop destruction was authorized by the U.S. government in late 1961 and terminated in 1971. Herbicides were also used to clear vegetation around military bases. Application of herbicides was accomplished primarily by the U.S. Air Force in aerial spraying using fixed-wing aircraft in Operation Ranch Hand. Army Chemical Corps personnel were responsible for smaller operations that included helicopter spraying as well as ground spraying using a variety of specialized and improvised equipment. Herbicides were probably also handled and used by other personnel, such as Navy riverine patrols and the engineering personnel who were responsible for constructing fire support bases (IOM, 1994).

Several different herbicides were used in Vietnam. Most were given designations (e.g., Orange, White, Pink) based on the color of the identification band on their storage drums. Listed in Table 1-2 are the most

INTRODUCTION AND BACKGROUND

TABLE 1-2 Herbicides Most Commonly Used in Vietnam

Herbicide	Principal Constituents	Dates of Use	Amount Sprayed (liters)
Pink	2,4,5-T	1961, 1965	50,312 (plus 413,852 in procurement records)
Green	2,4,5-T	1962–1964	31,026 (shown in procurement records)
Purple	2,4-D; 2,4,5-T	1962–1965	1,892,733
Orange	2,4-D; 2,4,5-T	1965–1970	45,677,937 (may include Orange II)
Orange II	2,4-D; 2,4,5-T	After 1968?	3,591,000 (minimum amount shipped)
White	2,4-D; picloram	1966–1971	20,556,525
Blue (powder)	Cacodylic acid; sodium cacodylate	1962–1964	25,650
Blue (aqueous solution)	Sodium cacodylate; cacodylic acid	1964–1971	4,715,731

NOTE: 2,4-D is 2,4-dichlorophenoxyacetic acid; 2,4,5-T is 2,4,5-trichlorophenoxyacetic acid. 2,4,5-T was contaminated with 2,3,7,8-tetrachlorodibenzo-p-dioxin (TCDD).
SOURCES: Adapted from Young et al., 1978; Stellman et al., 2003a; IOM, 2007.

commonly used herbicides, their principal constituents, their dates of use, and estimates of the amount sprayed. The principal defoliants were Agent Orange and Agent White, whereas crop destruction was often accomplished with Agent Blue.

The herbicide amounts in Table 1-2 were estimated from a combination of records on procurement, Ranch Hand spray missions and other operations, and disposal of surplus supplies (Young et al., 1978; Stellman et al., 2003a). The current estimates reflect the results of archival research, most recently by Stellman and colleagues (2003a), to assemble data from military records. Because Ranch Hand spray missions were subject to a formal high-level approval process, those records are considered to be relatively more complete than records of herbicide use in other contexts (e.g., perimeter spraying around military bases), which was authorized and managed by local commanders (IOM, 1994).

Emergence of Concerns About Potential Health Effects of Herbicides

The herbicides used in Vietnam were similar to products that had been in routine use in the United States and elsewhere for control of unwanted vegetation. In Vietnam, they were generally applied at a rate of 3 gallons per acre to maximize their effectiveness on tropical vegetation (Darrow et al., 1969). Lower application rates of 1 to 1.5 gallons per acre were considered effective for the vegetation types found in the United States (Department of the Army, 1971). By the end of the 1960s, however, concern had arisen that 2,4,5-T posed a hazard to human health. That concern contributed to a decision in 1970 to end the use in Vietnam of the herbicides that contained 2,4,5-T, and all official herbicide use ended in 1971. Remaining herbicide stocks were removed from Vietnam and subsequently destroyed.

Investigation had found that herbicides containing 2,4,5-T were contaminated with TCDD, an unwanted and highly toxic byproduct of the manufacturing process. This included Agent Orange, the herbicide used in greatest quantity in Vietnam, as well as agents Pink, Green, and Purple. In the 1970s, TCDD levels were measured in samples of the remaining stocks of these herbicides, but the TCDD levels found were not necessarily representative of the contamination levels of the herbicides applied in Vietnam. Furthermore, the TCDD contamination is thought to have varied over time and across manufacturing lots (Young et al., 1976).

During the 1970s, concern grew among Vietnam veterans and their families that the veterans were experiencing health problems because of exposure to herbicides in Vietnam, especially to the TCDD-contaminated Agent Orange. Claims for eligibility for health care services and disability compensation posed a challenge for VA: Information about the human health effects of herbicide and TCDD exposure was limited, and in most cases military service records provided no clear means to establish that a veteran had been exposed to an herbicide in Vietnam.

Studying Health Effects and Herbicide Exposure

Many different efforts have been pursued by Congress, federal agencies, and independent researchers to address the concerns about health effects that might result from herbicide exposure in Vietnam and to establish whether exposure occurred. In the early 1970s, for example, the National Academy of Sciences (NRC, 1974) conducted a broad congressionally mandated review of the effects of herbicide use in Vietnam, which included onsite investigations and initial construction of a computerized database on Ranch Hand spray missions (the HERBS tapes). By the end of the decade, the General Accounting Office (GAO, now named the Government Accountability Office) had investigated the potential for troops to be exposed to herbicides from Ranch Hand spraying (GAO, 1979). In 1979, the U.S. Air Force initiated a 20-year follow-up study of the health of Ranch Hand personnel (IOM, 2006), whose assignments meant both that they were in frequent proximity to herbicides and that their exposure history would not be representative of most troops who served in Vietnam.

VA and subsequently CDC were directed by Congress to conduct large epidemiologic studies of the health effects of herbicide exposure among the Vietnam veteran population, but these studies were never completed as planned, in part because of the lack of credible methods of determining herbicide exposure levels among veterans (e.g., CDC, 1988d; IOM, 1994). However, both VA and CDC completed other studies of the health of Vietnam veterans, many of which used service in Vietnam as a surrogate for herbicide exposure (e.g., Kang et al., 1986; Breslin et al., 1988; CDC, 1988a,b,c, 1990a,b,c; Watanabe and Kang, 1996; also see Appendix B).

In 1991, Public Law (P.L.) 102-4, known as the Agent Orange Act of 1991, established that Vietnam veterans with chloracne that developed within 1 year of leaving Vietnam, non-Hodgkin's lymphoma, or certain soft tissue sarcomas would be presumed to have been exposed to an herbicide in Vietnam and therefore be eligible for disability compensation.

Among its other provisions, P.L. 102-4 also directed VA to contract with the National Academy of Sciences to conduct biennial reviews of the published scientific literature to assess the strength of the evidence regarding associations between exposure to herbicides (or specific constituent chemical compounds) used in Vietnam and health outcomes of concern. To date seven reviews have been published (IOM, 1994, 1996, 1999, 2001, 2003c, 2005, 2007).[2] These reviews include consideration of evidence from available studies of Vietnam veterans, but they rely more heavily on studies of other populations, especially chemical production and agricultural workers as well as community residents exposed through environmental contamination, including industrial accidents. As directed by P.L. 102-4 (and reauthorized in P.L. 107-103), VA has used the findings from these reviews to designate additional health conditions as presumed to have a connection to military service in Vietnam (see Table 1-3). The IOM findings and the VA decisions on presumptive connections to military service are all based on evidence of statistical associations between health effects and herbicide exposure, not on evidence that is necessarily strong enough to demonstrate a causal relationship.

The Current Study

Congress originally sought from the IOM reviews an assessment of the increased risk that Vietnam veterans would have for conditions found to be associated with herbicide exposure. None of the review committees have been able to make quantitative assessments of this risk, in part, because credible direct or proxy measurements of Vietnam veterans' herbicide exposure have not been available.

---

[2]In addition to these broad reviews, IOM committees have also conducted reviews for specific health outcomes (IOM, 2000, 2002, 2004).

TABLE 1-3 Conditions Designated by the Department of Veterans Affairs as Presumed to Have Resulted from Exposure to Herbicides Used in Vietnam

• Acute and subacute peripheral neuropathy	• Prostate cancer
• Chloracne	• Respiratory cancers
• Chronic lymphocytic leukemia	(lung, bronchus, larynx, and trachea)
• Hodgkin's disease	• Soft-tissue sarcoma, acute
• Multiple myeloma	• Spina bifida in offspring of Vietnam veterans
• Non-Hodgkin's lymphoma	• Type II diabetes mellitus
• Porphyria cutanea tarda	

SOURCE: VA, 2007.

The first of the biennial reviews included a recommendation that this problem be addressed by an attempt to develop an exposure reconstruction model that could be considered valid for use in epidemiologic studies of veterans (IOM, 1994). VA responded to this recommendation by commissioning the IOM to assess the scientific issues that a research proposal would need to address, oversee the selection of a contractor to conduct the work, monitor progress during the course of the contract, and evaluate the product produced by the contractor (IOM, 1997, 2003a,b). The contract for the work was awarded in 1998 to researchers at the Columbia University Mailman School of Public Health (Jeanne Mager Stellman, Ph.D., principal investigator).

The project resulted in the development of a software tool called the Herbicide Exposure Assessment–Vietnam (HEA-V). The HEA-V uses a geographic information system (GIS) to link computerized databases containing information on the timing, amount, and locations of herbicide spraying with data on troop locations over time to calculate two metrics—"hits" and an exposure opportunity index (EOI)—representing exposure (HEA-V, 2003; Stellman and Stellman, 2003; Stellman et al., 2003b). These metrics are designed to serve as proxies for herbicide exposure. They account for differences in exposure that are likely to result from differences among individuals or units in their proximity in time and space to sprayed locations. The software and related databases are discussed in more detail in Chapter 2.

With the software and databases in hand, VA returned to the IOM for guidance on their use. In a presentation to the committee (Brown, 2007), VA's interests were described as including obtaining advice on effective use of the model in studies of illnesses previously associated with herbicide exposure and on the usefulness of existing information on Vietnam veterans who have died or who have certain diseases. VA was also interested in

ISSUES IN ASSESSING HERBICIDE EXPOSURE IN VIETNAM FOR EPIDEMIOLOGIC STUDIES

The committee identified four considerations as being central to its task. First, it was essential to be clear about the nature of the exposure assessment model and what it does and does not claim to do. The committee approached the model as a means of generating a quantitative representation of *opportunity* for herbicide exposure, not actual environmental levels, personal exposure levels, or biological dose levels. Although direct measurement of individual doses or exposure levels is the ideal, many studies of environmental and occupational health hazards must rely on proxy measures similar in concept to the direct hits metric or the EOI metric produced by the Stellman team's model (i.e., inferred exposure based on spatial and temporal proximity of the persons at risk to a source of the agent), as discussed in Chapter 3. For example, location of residence has been used as a proxy for exposure to ambient air pollution, recognizing that there will nonetheless be variation in individual exposure depending on factors such as the indoor environment and time–activity patterns (e.g., Briggs, 2003; Colvile et al., 2003).

Second, the committee gave careful consideration to the information needed to use the model. This included gaining an understanding of strengths and limitations of data on herbicide spraying, troop locations, and health outcomes. Issues of access to and usability of these data were also important. The committee notes that although attention in past studies has often focused on TCDD, the spraying database includes information on all herbicides for which records were available, and the committee made its assessment from this broader perspective.

Third, the committee considered the feasibility of a validation study to determine whether the metrics produced ("direct hits" and EOI) and the tools used to generate them "worked," that is, whether they locate spraying and troops accurately (opportunity for exposure) and whether doing so is related to actual exposure (through comparisons with other sources of information on exposure, such as blood levels or environmental samples). The goal of environmental epidemiology is the assessment of associations between exposure to a substance in the environment and a health outcome of interest. Research often advances through successive approximations of exposure, so that the utility of the model is defined in part by the methods it improves upon and does not depend solely on how closely the model approaches absolute accuracy.

Fourth, with the nature of the model and its metrics clearly in mind, the committee considered the potential contributions and pitfalls from using it in epidemiologic studies. Of particular interest in those deliberations were the potential to study Vietnam veterans directly, the degree to which exposure classification might be improved if the model was to be used, and the appropriate interpretation of the results of any such studies.

THE COMMITTEE'S REPORT

The remainder of the report presents the committee's findings and conclusions concerning use of the exposure assessment model and the committee's recommendations regarding epidemiologic studies that might be considered. Chapter 2 reviews the essential features of the model developed by the Stellman team. Chapter 3 presents the committee's assessment of the model within the context of an exposure hierarchy, with a review of key components of the model and the measures of exposure opportunity that the model can generate. Chapter 4 discusses the accessibility of data on military units and personnel needed to conduct studies using the model. Chapter 5 concludes the report with the committee's assessment of and recommendations concerning the development of epidemiologic studies that incorporate use of the exposure assessment model.

REFERENCES

Breslin, P., H. K. Kang, Y. Lee, V. Burt, and B. Shepard. 1988. Proportionate mortality study of US Army and US Marine Corps veterans of the Vietnam War. *Journal of Occupational Medicine* 30(5):412–419.

Briggs, D. 2003. Environmental measurement and modeling: Geographical information systems. In *Exposure assessment in occupational and environmental epidemiology*, edited by M. J. Nieuwenhuijsen. New York: Oxford University Press.

Brown, M. 2007. *Charge to the NAS/IOM Committee on Making Best Use of the Agent Orange Exposure Reconstruction Model*. Written comments submitted to the Committee on Making Best Use of the Agent Orange Exposure Reconstruction Model, Meeting 1, March 8, Washington, DC.

CDC (Centers for Disease Control and Prevention). 1988a. Health status of Vietnam veterans: I. Psychosocial characteristics. *Journal of the American Medical Association* 259(18):2701–2707.

CDC. 1988b. Health status of Vietnam veterans: II. Physical health. *Journal of the American Medical Association* 259(18):2708–2714.

CDC. 1988c. Health status of Vietnam veterans: III. Reproductive outcomes and child health. *Journal of the American Medical Association* 259(18):2715–2719.

CDC. 1988d. Serum 2,3,7,8-tetrachlorodibenzo-p-dioxin levels in U.S. Army Vietnam-era veterans. *Journal of the American Medical Association* 260(9):1249–1254.

CDC. 1990a. The association of selected cancers with service in the U.S. military in Vietnam: I. Non-Hodgkin's lymphoma. *Archives of Internal Medicine* 150:2473–2483.

CDC. 1990b. The association of selected cancers with service in the U.S. military in Vietnam: II. Soft-tissue and other sarcomas. *Archives of Internal Medicine* 150:2485–2492.

CDC. 1990c. The association of selected cancers with service in the U.S. military in Vietnam: III. Hodgkin's disease, nasal cancer, nasopharyngeal cancer, and primary liver cancer. *Archives of Internal Medicine* 150:2495–2505.

Colvile, R., D. Briggs, and M. J. Nieuwenhuijsen. 2003. Environmental measurement and modeling: Introduction and source dispersion modeling. In *Exposure assessment in occupational and environmental epidemiology*, edited by M. J. Nieuwenhuijsen. New York: Oxford University Press.

Darrow, R. A., K. R. Irish, and C. E. Hinarik. 1969. *Herbicides used in Southeast Asia*. Technical Report SAOQ-TR-69-11078. Fort Detrick, MD: U.S. Army Plant Sciences Laboratories.

Department of the Army. 1971. *Tactical employment of herbicides*. Field Manual FM 3-3. Washington, DC: Department of the Army.

DePue, M. 2006. Vietnam War: The individual rotation policy. *Vietnam Magazine*. http://www.historynet.com/magazines/vietnam/4632961.html (accessed September 20, 2007).

DoD (U.S. Department of Defense). 2007. *Military personnel historical reports*. http://siadapp.dmdc.osd.mil/personnel/MILITARY/history/309hist.htm (accessed August 2, 2007).

GAO (General Accounting Office). 1979. *U.S. ground troops in South Vietnam were in areas sprayed with Herbicide Orange*. FPCD-80-23. Washington, DC: U.S. Government Printing Office.

HEA-V (Herbicide Exposure Assessment–Vietnam). 2003. *CD-ROM, version 1.0.2. Software and accompanying electronic documentation*. New York: Columbia University.

IOM (Institute of Medicine). 1994. *Veterans and Agent Orange: Health effects of herbicides used in Vietnam*. Washington, DC: National Academy Press.

IOM. 1996. *Veterans and Agent Orange: Update 1996*. Washington, DC: National Academy Press.

IOM. 1997. *Characterizing exposure of veterans to Agent Orange and other herbicides used in Vietnam: Scientific considerations regarding a request for proposals for research*. Washington, DC: National Academy Press.

IOM. 1999. *Veterans and Agent Orange: Update 1998*. Washington, DC: National Academy Press.

IOM. 2000. *Veterans and Agent Orange: Herbicide/dioxin exposure and Type 2 diabetes*. Washington, DC: National Academy Press.

IOM. 2001. *Veterans and Agent Orange: Update 2000*. Washington, DC: National Academy Press.

IOM. 2002. *Veterans and Agent Orange: Herbicide/dioxin exposure and acute myelogenous leukemia in the children of Vietnam veterans*. Washington, DC: National Academy Press.

IOM. 2003a. *Characterizing exposure of veterans to Agent Orange and other herbicides used in Vietnam: Interim findings and recommendations*. Washington, DC: The National Academies Press.

IOM. 2003b. *Characterizing exposure of veterans to Agent Orange and other herbicides used in Vietnam: Final report*. Washington, DC: The National Academies Press.

IOM. 2003c. *Veterans and Agent Orange: Update 2002*. Washington, DC: The National Academies Press.

IOM. 2004. *Veterans and Agent Orange: Length of presumptive period for association between exposure and respiratory cancer*. Washington, DC: The National Academies Press.

IOM. 2005. *Veterans and Agent Orange: Update 2004*. Washington, DC: The National Academies Press.

IOM. 2006. *Disposition of the Air Force Health Study*. Washington, DC: The National Academies Press.

IOM. 2007. *Veterans and Agent Orange: Update 2006*. Washington, DC: The National Academies Press.

Kang, H. K. 2007. *Data resources within VA for an epidemiological study of Vietnam veterans*. PowerPoint presentation to the IOM Committee on Making Best Use of the Agent Orange Reconstruction Model, Meeting 2, April 30–May 1, Washington, DC.

Kang, H. K., L. Weatherbee, P. Breslin, Y. Lee, and B. Shepard. 1986. Soft tissue sarcomas and military service in Vietnam: A case comparison group analysis of hospital patients. *Journal of Occupational and Environmental Medicine* 28(12):1215–1218.

NRC (National Research Council). 1974. *The effects of herbicides in South Vietnam*. Washington, DC: National Academy of Sciences.

Stellman, J. M., and S. D. Stellman. 2003. *Contractor's final report: Characterizing exposure of veterans to Agent Orange and other herbicides in Vietnam*. Submitted to the National Academy of Sciences, Institute of Medicine, in fulfillment of Subcontract VA-5124-98-0019, June 30, 2003.

Stellman, S. D., and J. M. Stellman. 2004. Exposure opportunity models for Agent Orange, dioxin, and other military herbicides used in Vietnam, 1961–1971. *Journal of Exposure Analysis and Environmental Epidemiology* 14(4):354–362.

Stellman, J. M., S. D. Stellman, R. Christian, T. Weber, and C. Tomasallo. 2003a. The extent and patterns of usage of Agent Orange and other herbicides in Vietnam. *Nature* 422(6933):681–687.

Stellman, J. M., S. D. Stellman, T. Weber, C. Tomasallo, A. B. Stellman, and R. Christian, Jr. 2003b. A geographic information system for characterizing exposure to Agent Orange and other herbicides in Vietnam. *Environmental Health Perspectives* 111(3):321–328.

The U.S. Army in Vietnam: Background, buildup, and operations, 1950–1967. 2005. In *American military history, Volume II, The United States Army in a global era, 1917–2003*, edited by R. W. Stewart. Washington, DC: Center of Military History, United States Army. http://www.army.mil/cmh/books/AMH-V2/PDF/Chapter10.pdf (accessed September 20, 2007).

USMC (U.S. Marine Corps). 1985. *The Marines in Vietnam: 1954–1973*. Washington, DC: History and Museums Division, U.S. Marine Corps.

VA (U.S. Department of Veterans Affairs). 2007. *Vietnam veterans benefit from Agent Orange rules*. http://www.vba.va.gov/bln/21/benefits/herbicide/AOno1.htm (accessed July 9, 2007).

Watanabe, K. K., and H. K. Kang. 1996. Mortality patterns among Vietnam veterans. *Journal of Occupational and Environmental Medicine* 38(3):272–278.

Young, A. L., C. E. Thalken, E. L. Arnold, J. M. Cupello, and L. G. Cockerham. 1976. *Fate of 2,3,7,8-tetrachlorodibenzo-p-dioxin (TCDD) in the environment: Summary and decontamination recommendations*. USAFA-TR-76-18. Colorado Springs, CO: Department of Chemistry and Biological Sciences, USAF Academy.

Young, A. L., J. A. Calcagni, C. E. Thalken, and J. W. Tremblay. 1978. *The toxicology, environmental fate, and human risk of Herbicide Orange and its associated dioxin*. OEHL TR-78-92, Final Report. Brooks Air Force Base, TX: U.S. Air Force Occupational and Environmental Health Laboratory.

2

The Herbicide Exposure Assessment Model

In 2003 Jeanne Mager Stellman, Ph.D., and colleagues completed their project to develop methods to retrospectively characterize the exposure of Vietnam veterans to herbicides used by the military in Vietnam. The project resulted in the compilation of databases on herbicide spraying, the identification and location of certain military units, and the development of a software tool—Herbicide Exposure Assessment–Vietnam (HEA-V)—that facilitates use of an exposure assessment model to calculate two proximity-based herbicide exposure metrics: a "hits" measure and an exposure opportunity index (EOI) (Stellman and Stellman, 2003). The model and the HEA-V software tool use a geographic information system (GIS) that makes it possible to link an extensive database providing timing and location of herbicide application with the location histories of individuals or military units. The work was described in detail in a final report submitted to an Institute of Medicine committee overseeing the project and to the Department of Veterans Affairs (VA) (Stellman and Stellman, 2003). In addition, Stellman and colleagues published three peer-reviewed papers on various aspects of their work (Stellman et al., 2003a,b; Stellman and Stellman, 2004).

This chapter presents an overview of the exposure assessment concepts underlying measures of exposure opportunity and provides a brief summary of the Stellman team's exposure assessment model and the related software and databases as described in the final report to VA, the journal articles, and presentations by Dr. Stellman to the committee.

THE EXPOSURE OPPORTUNITY CONCEPT

Quantifying "exposure opportunity" refers to assessing the *potential* for exposure rather than assessing the exposure itself and thus is, at best, a crude approximation of toxicologic dose. Measures like the EOI are particularly useful in situations where historical data on body burden or environmental exposure concentrations are not available, and where measurements based on newly collected samples are not useful for estimating past exposures.

The Stellman team's two measures of exposure opportunity are based on presence at a location that records indicate was within a specified distance of herbicide spraying and can be considered surrogates of exposure. By contrast, many past studies of Vietnam veterans and their health status have used service in Vietnam—a marker even further removed from dose than the proximity-based measures—as an exposure surrogate (e.g., CDC, 1987; Breslin et al., 1988; Dalager and Kang, 1997; also see Appendix B). Because measurements of body burden, dose, or exposure concentrations are often not feasible in retrospective studies of occupational or environmental hazards, surrogate measures of potential for exposure (such as the opportunity index) are commonly used in studies of occupational and environmental hazards.

Exposure–Disease Pathway

It is often helpful to think of health effects that result from exposure to a toxic material in terms of a pathway from the introduction of the toxic material into the environment to the production of the health effects (Figure 2-1). Following the introduction of a toxic material, processes that affect the fate and transport of the material lead to its presence in varying concentrations across the environment. Contact between people and the toxic substance—modified by individual behaviors—can lead to exposure via three principal routes: inhalation, dermal exposure, or ingestion. Pharmacokinetic processes then govern the concentration of the toxic substance and its metabolites in the body, including at the target organ. The factors determining the biologically effective dose can depend on the health effect of interest. For example, for some diseases cumulative dose might be important, while for others the peak dose may be the most relevant consideration. Timing of the dose can also be critical. For cancer, relevant doses may occur decades prior to diagnosis; for developmental effects, the relevant exposure of the developing organism can occur during specific time windows (e.g., early in pregnancy).

THE HERBICIDE EXPOSURE ASSESSMENT MODEL 27

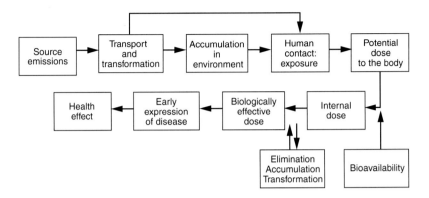

FIGURE 2-1 Pathway from emission of a contaminant to a health effect.
SOURCE: Reprinted with permission from Lioy, 1990. Copyright 1990 American Chemical Society.

Exposure Assessment Hierarchy

The pathway notion provides a useful conceptual structure for thinking about the relationship between exposure and outcome, but the practicalities of actually doing a study must also be considered. For example, while the pathway diagram suggests that biomarkers (which reflect internal dose in Figure 2-1) can provide an exposure measure that is close to ideal, such measures may not be practical if no biomarker has been identified for the compound under study or if, in a retrospective study, too much time has elapsed between exposure and measurement for a biomarker to be detected. Thus, when designing or evaluating studies, it is useful to keep in mind the types of data associated with the exposure assessment hierarchy (Table 2-1). Although it was developed in the context of community exposures to hazardous waste sites, it has wider applicability (Nieuwenhuijsen, 2003).

The idea behind the exposure assessment hierarchy is that for any given study there exists a range of possible exposure metrics that vary in accuracy. Quantified personal measurements—such as exposure biomarkers or personal air monitoring—generally provide the best data if they are biologically relevant. Beyond that, various increasingly indirect exposure metrics are possible. For example, such measures may be based on combinations of ambient environmental measurements and individual-level information on behavior patterns that affect exposure; estimates of ambient environmental concentrations derived from fate and transport modeling; or distance and

TABLE 2-1 Data for a Hierarchy of Exposure Assessment

Types of Data	Approximation to Actual Exposure
1. Residence or employment in defined geographical area (e.g., a county) of the site	Poorest
2. Residence or employment in geographic area in reasonable proximity to site where exposure can be assumed	
3. Distance from site or duration of residence in area	
4. Distance from site and duration of residence	
5. Quantified surrogates of exposure (e.g., estimates of drinking water use)	
6. Quantified area or ambient measurements in the vicinity of the residence or other sites of activity	
7. Quantified personal measurements	Best

SOURCE: Adapted from NRC, 1991.

duration, in combination or separately, as surrogates for fate and transport modeling. The poorest exposure approximation in the hierarchy is residence or employment in the same area (e.g., a county) as the exposure source.

Despite their limitations, such relatively crude exposure surrogates as location have been used effectively in many environmental and occupational health studies. Indeed, geographic approaches to exposure assessment can be especially useful when pollutants vary significantly over space in a systematic manner (Briggs, 2003; Colvile et al., 2003).

Several considerations are important when thinking about the hierarchy. If there is a relationship between exposure and outcome, for instance, more accurate measures of exposure often tend to provide a better ability to detect effects. This occurs because errors in exposure measurement tend to diminish estimated effects if the errors are non-differential, that is, if they do not depend on the outcome. Although there are exceptions, this holds true in many important cases, such as the regression analysis of a continuous exposure measure with random measurement error. On the other hand, while it is nearly always possible to imagine better exposure measures, additional details do not always dramatically improve results. For example, if personal behaviors relevant for exposure do not differ much between individuals, then adding information on those behaviors will not change the rank order of exposure very much (e.g., Vieira et al., 2005).

COMPONENTS OF THE HERBICIDE EXPOSURE ASSESSMENT MODEL

The exposure assessment model developed by the Stellman team brings together several components. The GIS provides a method for linking detailed data on the location of herbicide spraying with data on the location of military personnel or military units or facilities and can also be applied to Vietnamese communities or residents. The GIS relies on a detailed base map of Vietnam, a database for herbicide spraying missions, and software that can calculate exposure opportunity measures (both direct hits and cumulative exposure opportunity) based on entered locations. Also available is a database that assigns a soil type to each grid cell in the GIS.

In the GIS, Vietnam is portioned into a grid with the smallest unit being a rectangle of 0.01° of latitude by 0.01° of longitude, which is approximately 1.2 square kilometers. The center point of each of these cells is the reference location for all of the positions within that grid cell. As a result, the grid cell size defines the ultimate spatial resolution of the GIS.

The Stellman team has also done extensive work to compile databases on the identification of military units that served in Vietnam and on the location of many units during the period herbicide spraying took place. Data on the location of military units or on the personnel who served in them are essential inputs for generating unit- or person-level exposure opportunity scores, but unlike the geographic parameters or the data on herbicide spraying, these databases are not contained in the herbicide exposure assessment software.

Each of these components is discussed in the sections that follow.

Measures of Exposure Opportunity

The exposure opportunity assessment model described here and discussed throughout this report is an extension and refinement of earlier approaches developed by the Stellman team (Stellman and Stellman, 1986; Stellman et al., 1988) to produce quantitative surrogates of exposure that take into account proximity in time and space to herbicide spraying over a specific period during the war in Vietnam. Two types of measures of exposure opportunity can be generated with the current GIS and software.

One measure provides the number of "hits," or instances of a herbicide spray application, that occurred within a certain distance (0.5 km, 1 km, 2 km, or 5 km) of a given grid location (Figure 2-2).

The second measure, EOI, takes into account the potential exposure from past as well as same-day spraying. The Stellman team refers to the

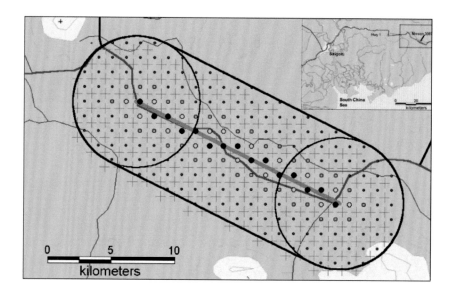

FIGURE 2-2 Region of Vietnam approximately 80 kilometers east of Saigon (see inset), showing the flight path of Ranch Hand mission no. 3087, flown on May 11, 1967, (straight orange line) along Highway 1 (jagged red line). The GIS grid system is shown as horizontal and vertical lines spaced 0.01° apart. Contained within a 5-kilometer buffer drawn around the flight path (heavy black line) are the centroids of the 210 cells that fell within 5 kilometers of the flight path, with size and color indicating proximity to the defoliation flight path: large black circles = 0.5 kilometer or less; large open circles = 0.5–1 kilometer; small shaded squares = 1–2 kilometers; small black circles = 2–5 kilometers.
SOURCE: Stellman and Stellman, 2004. Reprinted by permission from Macmillan Publishers Ltd: *Journal of Exposure Analysis and Environmental Epidemiology* 14:354–362, Copyright 2004.

possibility of exposure to residual herbicide from sprays on prior days as "indirect exposure." To calculate the combined direct and indirect EOI, their model takes into account for each spraying mission the quantity of herbicide or concentration factor; the reciprocal distance of the exposure location from the herbicide spray; a time factor, chosen to be a first-order environmental decay of the sprayed herbicide over time; and the concept of continuous dispersion of herbicide all along the path of the flight.

The EOI developed and refined by the Stellman team is reported to be quantitative on a ratio scale, meaning that an EOI of 1,000 indicates twice as much exposure opportunity as an EOI of 500 (Stellman et al., 2003b).

However, given that the EOI is a measure of exposure opportunity, not actual exposure, the EOI is not necessarily proportional to the dose of herbicide that an exposed individual would have received.

Software System Automating Exposure Opportunity Calculations

The HEA-V software (HEA-V, 2003) was developed to facilitate and automate the calculations involved in assessing proximity to the herbicide spraying that is known to have occurred during the Vietnam War. The software, which is accompanied by a manual to guide users, prompts users to provide—either in a file that can be imported or by directly entering the data—the information needed to calculate hits or an EOI for individuals or military units of interest. The necessary inputs include the longitude and latitude for each of the individuals' or units' locations during a period of interest and the start and end dates for their presence at each of these locations.

After the necessary inputs have been provided, the software allows users to make a series of decisions regarding the nature of the analysis sought. For example, a user may specify that hits or EOI scores be calculated for only one kind of herbicide or one type of spraying (e.g., fixed-wing aircraft versus helicopter). Users can also designate the half-life for environmental decay of the agent of interest, or limit the locations, dates, or gallonage (the quantity of herbicide for a spray mission) to be considered. The software also aids in the selection of preferred outputs and in the documentation of analyses.

The Herbicide Spray Database

The herbicide exposure assessment model incorporates a database with detailed information on the timing and locations of herbicide applications. The file contains information for 9,141 spray missions, 65 percent of which were conducted by the U.S. Air Force using C-123 fixed-wing aircraft as part of Operation Ranch Hand. A review of the database showed that these Ranch Hand missions delivered 95 percent of the total amount of herbicide recorded as dispersed by the U.S. military in Vietnam. The remaining 35 percent of missions recorded in the database were U.S. Army helicopter and ground spraying activities or missions with an unspecified delivery method. Records of helicopter missions were kept with the fixed wing records beginning in 1968, but ground spraying was not tracked as part of a permanent record system (Stanton, 1989).

To assemble these data, Dr. Stellman's team has described drawing on Department of Defense (DoD) files known as HERBS and Services HERBS; extensive research into military records held by the National Archives and Records Administration; and assistance from the Army's Center for Research of Unit Records (CRUR; now the Joint Services Records Research Center, JSRRC) (Stellman and Stellman, 2003).[1] This work was the basis for the elimination of duplicate records, the addition of records for some previously undocumented missions, and the correction of or addition of missing information to some other records.

The HERBS and Services HERBS data use the DoD's version of the UTM coordinate system to represent the location of herbicide spraying missions. UTM refers to the Universal Transverse Mercator map projection, for which latitude and longitude are transformed into meter distances on a projection of the earth's surface onto thin strips running from pole to pole. DoD's version of UTM consists of a two-letter code identifying a particular 100,000-by-100,000-meter grid cell within the map, followed by two three-digit sequences indicating the distance in hundreds of meters east and north, respectively, from the southwest corner of the grid cell. Although the UTM coordinates have a nominal precision of 100 meters, it was difficult for aircrews and ground troops to determine locations with that level of accuracy (Young et al., 2004).

Spraying mission flight paths are denoted by a sequence of linear legs between UTM coordinates. The Stellman team converted these UTM coordinates into longitude and latitude using software from what is now the National Geospatial-Intelligence Agency (Stellman, 2007) and placed flight paths onto their GIS's grid defined by the 0.01°-by-0.01° cells mentioned above (approximately 1.2 km^2).

UNIT LOCATION INFORMATION

To use the GIS and exposure assessment model to estimate veterans' potential exposure to herbicides, coordinates indicating location are needed for each day that a study subject was present in Vietnam (or for a specific period of Vietnam service). Locations of individual service members in Vietnam were not recorded, so the recorded locations of the military units in which they served are used to impute the locations of individuals.

The Stellman team has drawn upon a variety of sources to compile a comprehensive list of units that served in Vietnam. This list exists as a

---

[1] The Army unit currently designated as the U.S. Army and Joint Services Records Research Center (JSRRC) has operated under various other designations in the past, including the Environmental Support Group (ESG, 1980–1996), the Center for Research of Unit Records (CRUR, 1996–1998), and the Center for Unit Records Research (CURR, 1998–2006) (Hakenson, 2007). The principal responsibility of JSRRC and its predecessor organizations is to research military records to provide information related to veterans' claims filed with VA. JSRRC responds to requests from individual veterans, veterans service organizations, and VA. This report generally refers to the unit by its current designation of JSRRC.

database called UICLIST, which is independent of the herbicide exposure assessment software. Based upon units' missions, the Stellman team categorized them as stable (units whose missions did not require field maneuvers), mobile (units whose missions required leaving main base camps), or containing mobile elements within an otherwise stable unit. They have gathered location information on many stable units, including nearly all the combat arms support and combat support units assigned to Vietnam. They estimate that these units constitute about 80 percent of the Army troops who served in Vietnam (Stellman and Stellman, 2003). In addition to the data on these stable units, the Stellmans also have created a database capturing location information collected by JSRRC on Army combat battalions serving in the III Corps Tactical Zone during the years 1966–1969, a place and time of intense aerial herbicide spraying (Stellman et al., 2003a). Although the Stellman team has collected location information for many of the stable units in Vietnam and some of the combat units, it is likely that additional information on unit locations will have to be assembled for at least some of the participants in an epidemiologic study. The considerations involved in such efforts are discussed in Chapter 4.

It is important to note that the model is not applicable to Air Force Ranch Hand personnel and Army Chemical Corps personnel, whose exposures to herbicides are likely to be the highest of all veterans. Their herbicide exposures were primarily a direct result of duties that required handling or applying herbicides. By contrast, the model is designed to assess the exposure opportunity that would result from unintended proximity to herbicide spraying.

REFERENCES

Breslin, P., H. K. Kang, Y. Lee, V. Burt, and B. Shepard. 1988. Proportionate mortality study of US Army and US Marine Corps veterans of the Vietnam War. *Journal of Occupational Medicine* 30(5):412–419.

Briggs, D. 2003. Environmental measurement and modeling: Geographical information systems. In *Exposure assessment in occupational and environmental epidemiology*, edited by M. J. Nieuwenhuijsen. New York: Oxford University Press.

CDC (Centers for Disease Control and Prevention). 1987. Postservice mortality among Vietnam veterans. *Journal of the American Medical Association* 257(6):790–795.

Colvile, R., D. Briggs, and M. J. Nieuwenhuijsen. 2003. Environmental measurement and modeling: Introduction and source dispersion modeling. In *Exposure assessment in occupational and environmental epidemiology*, edited by M. J. Nieuwenhuijsen. New York: Oxford University Press.

Dalager, N. A., and H. K. Kang. 1997. Mortality among Army Chemical Corps Vietnam veterans. *American Journal of Industrial Medicine* 31:719–726.

Hakenson, D. 2007. Help with some names and dates? E-mail to L. Joellenbeck, Institute of Medicine, October 16.

HEA-V (Herbicide Exposure Assessment–Vietnam). 2003. *CD-ROM, version 1.0.2. Software and accompanying electronic documentation.* New York: Columbia University.

Lioy, P. J. 1990. Assessing total human exposure to contaminants: A multidisciplinary approach. *Environmental Science and Technology* 24(7):938–945.

Nieuwenhuijsen, M. J. 2003. Introduction to exposure assessment. In *Exposure assessment in occupational and environmental epidemiology*, edited by M. J. Nieuwenhuijsen. New York: Oxford University Press.

NRC (National Research Council). 1991. *Environmental epidemiology, Volume 1: Public health and hazardous wastes*. Washington, DC: National Academy Press.

Stanton, S. L. 1989. Area-scoring methodology for estimating Agent Orange exposure status of U.S. Army personnel in the Republic of Vietnam. In *Comparison of serum levels of 2,3,7,8-tetrachlorodibenzo-p-dioxin with indirect estimates of Agent Orange exposure among Vietnam veterans*, by Centers for Disease Control and Prevention. Atlanta, GA: Centers for Disease Control and Prevention.

Stellman, J. M. 2007. *Responses to IOM 091407*. Unpublished document submitted to the IOM Committee on Making the Best Use of the Agent Orange Reconstruction Model, September 14.

Stellman, S. D., and J. M. Stellman. 1986. Estimation of exposure to Agent Orange and other defoliants among American troops in Vietnam: A methodological approach. *American Journal of Industrial Medicine* 9(4):305–321.

Stellman, J. M., and S. D. Stellman. 2003. *Contractor's final report: Characterizing exposure of veterans to Agent Orange and other herbicides in Vietnam*. Submitted to the National Academy of Sciences, Institute of Medicine, in fulfillment of Subcontract VA-5124-98-0019, June 30, 2003.

Stellman, S. D., and J. M. Stellman. 2004. Exposure opportunity models for Agent Orange, dioxin, and other military herbicides used in Vietnam, 1961–1971. *Journal of Exposure Analysis and Environmental Epidemiology* 14:354–362.

Stellman, S. D., J. M. Stellman, and J. F. Sommer, Jr. 1988. Combat and herbicide exposures in Vietnam among a sample of American Legionnaires. *Environmental Research* 47:112–128.

Stellman, J. M., S. D. Stellman, R. Christian, T. Weber, and C. Tomasallo. 2003a. The extent and patterns of usage of Agent Orange and other herbicides in Vietnam. *Nature* 422:681–687.

Stellman, J. M., S. D. Stellman, T. Weber, C. Tomasallo, A. B. Stellman, and R. Christian, Jr. 2003b. A geographic information system for characterizing exposure to Agent Orange and other herbicides in Vietnam. *Environmental Health Perspectives* 111:321–328.

Vieira, V., A. Aschengrau, and D. Ozonoff. 2005. Impact of tetrachloroethylene-contaminated drinking water on the risk of breast cancer: Using a dose model to assess exposure in a case-control study. *Environmental Health* 4(1):3. http://www.ehjournal.net/content/4/1/3 (accessed August 7, 2007).

Young, A. L., P. F. Cecil, and J. F. Guilmartin, Jr. 2004. Assessing possible exposure of ground troops to Agent Orange during the Vietnam War: The use of contemporary military records. *Environmental Science and Pollution Research* 11(6):349–358.

3

Assessment of the Model and Its Capacity to Produce Useful Exposure Metrics

The central question before the committee was how the Stellman team's model for generating herbicide exposure opportunity metrics might best be used in epidemiologic studies of the health of Vietnam veterans. Before addressing that question, the committee judged it appropriate to first assess the strengths and weaknesses of the data and the calculations that are the basis for the Stellman team's exposure metrics and the infrastructure of their Herbicide Exposure Assessment–Vietnam (HEA-V) software tool. In this chapter, the committee elaborates on the concept of an exposure assessment hierarchy, as introduced in Chapter 2, to serve as the context for its assessment of the Stellman team's model. The chapter then focuses on (1) the data on geography and herbicide spraying that are the basic infrastructure of the model, (2) the exposure metrics—"hits" and an exposure opportunity index (EOI)—that the HEA-V helps to calculate, and (3) potential refinements of the model. The chapter also addresses concerns that have been raised about some aspects of the data and assumptions on herbicide spraying and the environmental fate and transport of the herbicides.

Use of the model in epidemiologic studies will require researchers to supply data on troop location histories and veterans' health outcomes. The committee's examination of these types of data and their acquisition is discussed in Chapter 4.

AN EXPOSURE ASSESSMENT HIERARCHY FOR VIETNAM VETERANS

The Stellman team has developed a geographic information system (GIS) for use in estimating herbicide exposure in Vietnam, and they have also developed the HEA-V, a computerized database engine that facilitates the linking of disparate georeferenced data and the calculation of exposure metrics (HEA-V, 2003). To understand the strengths and limitations of this approach for measuring the opportunity for herbicide exposure, the committee viewed the model in the context of an exposure assessment hierarchy.

Placing the Stellman Team's Model in an Exposure Assessment Hierarchy

As noted in Chapter 2, an exposure assessment hierarchy can help illustrate both the relationship between an environmental exposure and a health outcome and the levels at which "exposure" might be measured with greater or lesser accuracy. More specifically, Figure 3-1 illustrates the exposure assessment hierarchy that the committee used to guide its thinking on herbicide spraying in Vietnam and the level at which the Stellman team's model operates.

The simplest marker of exposure opportunity is presence or absence of a veteran in Vietnam (level 1). Level 2 uses information on proximity to spraying in space and time for military units or individuals. This is primarily the level at which the Stellman team's model operates. The exposure opportunity metrics of hits and EOIs are calculated for geographic locations, and those results can be combined with user-supplied information on the location histories of military units or personnel to calculate hits and EOIs at the unit or person level. A unit-level measurement would in effect assign the same EOI to all individuals within the unit. Hits and EOIs can be considered to serve as proximity-based surrogates of exposure.

The proximity-based exposure metrics might be refined by the incorporation of fate and transport models that provide estimates of the concentration of an herbicide in various environmental media (level 3). For example, a spray drift model or estimates of the proportion of the sprayed herbicide that reaches ground level might be used instead of proximity alone. The next level of refinement in estimating exposure (level 4) would require data on individual-level interactions with the environment (e.g., dermal exposure to soil, consumption of local food) to better estimate personal exposures and permit examination of differences among units or individuals present at the same places and times.

At the most highly refined level (level 5), information on pharmacokinetics—which relates to the body's absorption, distribution, metabolism, and elimina-

ASSESSMENT OF THE MODEL

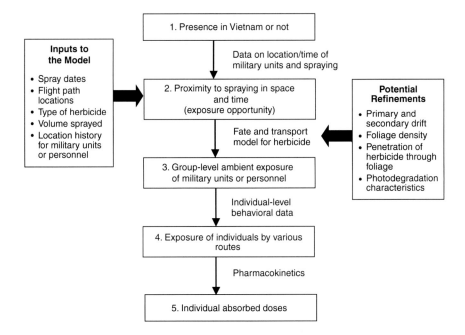

FIGURE 3-1 An exposure assessment hierarchy showing levels at which herbicide exposure in Vietnam can be assessed. The box on the left shows the inputs to the Stellman team's model, and the box on the right shows some potential inputs if a revised model were to incorporate fate and transport phenomena.

tion of chemicals—would be needed to estimate the doses of a toxic compound that individuals receive. Thus advancing through the hierarchy moves closer to measures of a truly biologically relevant dose. TCDD (2,3,7,8-tetrachlorodibenzo-p-dioxin) levels in serum or tissue have been used as biomarkers of exposure to the TCDD contaminant in Agent Orange and some of the other herbicides used in Vietnam, but comparable biomarkers are not available for any of the herbicides per se, and the usefulness of TCDD levels has receded as the time since exposure in Vietnam has increased.

Proximity-Based Surrogates of Exposure in Vietnam

The exposure assessment hierarchy is instructive in comparing the exposure metrics generated by the Stellman team's model and the exposure assessments used in previous epidemiologic studies of Vietnam veterans.

(See Appendix B for a table summarizing the exposure assessments used in studies of U.S. Vietnam veterans.) In most cases, military personnel were considered "exposed," not necessarily to herbicides but to the "war experience in total," if they were present in Vietnam during designated years or were part of specific military units at the division or corps level. In several studies, veterans' self-reports of herbicide exposure were used as the exposure metric. A few studies have included an effort to assess the location of study participants in relation to recorded herbicide spray locations. More detailed exposure assessments, including serum TCDD measurements, have been made for those military personnel who were part of the Operation Ranch Hand units or the Army Chemical Corps, both of which applied herbicides in Vietnam.

Proximity-based exposure metrics similar to those developed by the Stellman team were used in a 1986 validation study conducted in conjunction with the planning for a large Agent Orange Exposure Study to be done by the Centers for Disease Control and Prevention (CDC, 1989). The CDC "hits" metric defined an exposure hit as a unit's presence within 2 kilometers of spraying that occurred within the previous 6 days. CDC also developed a weighted hit score for which the weight was related to the environmental half-life of TCDD. The result was that troops within 2 kilometers of a spray path 1 day after spraying were assigned a higher exposure score than troops in the same location 5 days after spraying. Finally, CDC developed an "area score," which was based on the number of days a company was in one of five large, heavily sprayed regions of the III Corps Tactical Zone during 1967–1968 (CDC, 1989).

Other Uses of Proximity to Source as a Surrogate for Exposure

In environmental health studies, it is often necessary to make a retrospective assessment of a study population's exposures to an agent of interest. When stronger data, such as biomarker measurements for individuals or ambient environmental levels of an agent are unavailable, proximity to the agent has been used as an exposure surrogate. Such studies provide some insight into the usefulness of proximity as an exposure metric for herbicide use in Vietnam.

Seveso

Studies of the health effects of TCDD exposure from the 1976 industrial accident in Seveso, Italy, offer one example of a proximity-based approach to exposure assessment. Subjects were assigned to exposure zones based on the location of their homes, and these exposure zones were defined by proximity to the plant and measurements of surface soil contamination (Caramaschi et al., 1981). These environmental measurement-based exposure zones were associated with rates of chloracne, diabetes, and lymphatic and hematopoetic cancers (Bertazzi et al., 2001). They have also been correlated with serum TCDD levels on the basis of blood samples collected after the accident in 1976 and, later, in the 1990s, with serum TCDD concentrations being much higher on average in residents of the more highly exposed areas (e.g., Bertazzi et al., 1998; Eskenazi et al., 2004).

Agricultural Studies

Proximity to the locations of pesticide applications has also been explored as a potential surrogate for exposure in several U.S. studies. In an area of orchard cultivation in Washington State, organophosphate insecticide levels in carpet dust and metabolites in urine of children in agricultural families increased with self-reported proximity of homes to crop fields (Lu et al., 2000). Another study of children residing in a similar area of the state found that concentrations of organophosphate insecticide metabolites in urine were not related to proximity to fields but increased during the pesticide application season compared with other times of the year (Koch et al., 2002).

In Iowa, over 90 percent of crop acreage (primarily corn and soybeans) is treated with one or more herbicides. Detections of agricultural herbicides and herbicide concentrations in house dust samples increased significantly with increasing acreages of corn or soybean fields within 750 meters of homes (Ward et al., 2006). However, the location of crop acreage within specific buffer distances of 100–500 meters did not explain significantly more of the variation in pesticide level than total acreage within 750 meters (Ward et al., 2006). Another study in Iowa (Curwin et al., 2005) found no relationship between agricultural herbicide and insecticide concentrations in house dust and self-reported proximity to crop fields in nonfarm households; distance was classified in quarter-mile increments, ranging from less than 0.25 miles to more than 1 mile.

INFRASTRUCTURE OF THE STELLMAN TEAM'S MODEL

In view of the merit of the Stellman team's proximity-based approach as a reasonable step toward more accurate herbicide exposure assessment, the committee reviewed the components that are the infrastructure of the GIS and the HEA-V software. Three integral databases store basic inputs on dates (filename: DATES), geography (GridPoints), and the data on herbicide spraying (HERBS).

Time and Geography

Time references are essential in the calculation of the exposure metrics. Each date from January 1, 1961, through December 31, 1975, has been assigned four unique integer values corresponding to its day, week, month, and year within that 15-year period. The integer values facilitate the date-related calculations.

As noted in Chapter 2, the model uses a GIS that is based on a grid that covers all of South Vietnam (as well as sprayed areas in Cambodia and Laos). The grid uses fixed intervals of 0.01° of latitude and longitude, which results in 176,060 cells of approximately 1.2 square kilometers each (Stellman and Stellman, 2003). The coordinates of the southwest corner of a cell serve as the reference point, and each cell is assigned a unique identification number in the GridPoints database. Calculations of distance are made from the centroid of a cell, which is reported as being no more than 800 meters from any of the cell's corners (Stellman and Stellman, 2003).

These two databases are straightforward tools and are subject to little potential error or uncertainty. The committee notes, however, that the location data in military records from the Vietnam era, such as those for spray missions or sites of military encampments, were recorded with map coordinates in a version of the Universal Transverse Mercator (UTM) system used by the military, rather than in coordinates of latitude and longitude. The UTM values were converted to latitude and longitude using software from what is now the National Geospatial-Intelligence Agency (Stellman, 2007).

Herbicide Spraying

The third integral data component in the GIS is the information that the Stellman team has assembled on herbicide spraying. The data elements of the HEA-V HERBS file include information on when and where each herbicide mission took place, how the mission was conducted (e.g., fixed-wing aircraft or other means), what herbicide was used, and how much herbicide was used. Of particular interest to the committee in thinking about generating exposure opportunity metrics were the nature and quality of the data on the location of spraying and the amount of herbicide applied.

Stellman and colleagues (2003a) have described assembling this database by cleaning, combining, and reconciling data on spraying from several sources, including records on Operation Ranch Hand missions and U.S. Army helicopter and ground spraying activities (sources known as the HERBS and Services HERBS tapes); newly identified data from the National Archives; and data relating to aborted missions, emergency dumps, leaks, crashes, and other herbicide releases that were not part of standard spraying missions. They report having examined and reconciled multiple versions of previously compiled data on Ranch Hand missions, original U.S. Air Force records that included Daily Air Activities Reports (DAARs), and the contents of Air Force "project folders," which could include maps, after-action reports, and other documentation of groups of spraying missions (Stellman and Stellman, 2003).

Mission Records

The HEA-V HERBS file contains information on 9,141 separate spraying missions, of which 5,957 (65 percent) are recorded as Ranch Hand flights by C-123 fixed-wing aircraft. Records of these missions are considered relatively complete, especially for 1965–1971, in part because of the formal, high-level approval process for those missions (U.S. Army, 1985; Stellman et al., 2003a; Young et al., 2004a).

Also included in the HEA-V file is what is recognized as incomplete information on U.S. Army helicopter and ground spraying activities (U.S. Army, 1985; Stanton, 1989; IOM, 1994). A review of the file showed that it has records for 2,108 helicopter missions and 446 missions that used ground spraying equipment. (The delivery method is not specified for the remaining 630 missions, 70 percent of which were recorded as being for perimeter spraying around base camps, fire bases, air bases, and other fixed military camps.) Records of helicopter missions were kept with Ranch Hand records beginning in 1968, but ground spraying was not tracked as part of a permanent record system (Stanton, 1989). Information on herbicide use by the U.S. Navy, U.S. Marine Corps, Vietnamese, and other allied forces is not known to be available. The Stellman team's comparisons of spraying records with procurement records show disparities in both directions—in some cases (e.g., Agent Pink) it would appear that more herbicide was procured than documentation shows was sprayed, while in others (e.g., Agent Purple) it appears that more was sprayed than surviving records would indicate was procured (Stellman and Stellman, 2004).

Location of Herbicide Spraying

The location data in the HEA-V HERBS database identify the mission's region (the Corps Tactical Zone, e.g., III Corps) and sometimes the province in which the mission originated. A review of the file showed that for approximately 99 percent of the fixed-wing missions, UTM coordinates are available for the starting and ending points of the mission and for intermediate points at which the flight path changed or the spray was turned on or off. About 50 percent of helicopter missions and 60 percent of ground spraying missions are represented by a single UTM coordinate.

The HEA-V system represents the flight path for a mission by straight lines between the known UTM points (Stellman and Stellman, 2003), but actual routes may have curved to follow the path of a target such as a road or waterway. The Stellman team reported plans to use information on the nature of target areas to impute more realistic flight paths (Stellman and Stellman, 2004), but this work has not yet been completed (Stellman, 2007).

The records also include the number of fixed-wing planes flown in a given mission: 4.6 percent of these missions were flown with one aircraft, 21 percent with two, 44 percent with three, 11 percent with four, and 19 percent with five or more planes. The number of planes flown on a mission is a factor in the size of the area sprayed. Although the current version of the HEA-V does not account for differences among missions in the total width of their flight paths, the Stellman team has explored ways in which the information might be incorporated (Stellman, 2007).

Herbicide Agents and Volume Estimates

The HEA-V HERBS database identifies the herbicide used in a mission and the amount dispensed (the "gallonage"). "Incidents" that would have affected the dispersal of herbicide (e.g., an aborted flight, leaks) are identified as well. The Stellman team (2003b) reported that Agent Orange accounted for 62 percent of the total documented volume of herbicide used (approximately 12 million out of 19.5 million gallons), with 28 percent being Agent White, 6 percent being Agent Blue, 3 percent being other known herbicides, and 1 percent unknown agents. Although Stellman and colleagues (2003a) discuss the amount and variability of the TCDD contamination that may have been present in some of these herbicides (discussed later in this chapter), the HEA-V data do not incorporate any explicit estimates of TCDD levels for individual spray missions.

The available records show that 95 percent of the herbicide used was applied via the missions flown by fixed-wing aircraft as part of Operation Ranch Hand (Stellman et al., 2003a). The Stellman team's database shows that, overall, data on the amount of herbicide used are missing for 781 (8.5 percent) of the missions. The data are missing for only 0.9 percent of fixed-wing missions but for 33 percent of ground spraying missions.

As with the data on the location of spraying, the information on the herbicide agents and volumes sprayed appears to reflect the Stellman team's review of multiple sources, including attempts to reconcile herbicide procurement records with records of use and destruction of remaining stocks of these products (Stellman et al., 2003a). The magnitude of a separate set of volume estimates that were based on procurement and disposition records for 1965–1971 (17.4 million gallons of agents Orange, White, and Blue combined) (see Young et al., 1978) is similar to the amount in the Stellman team's data drawn from Ranch Hand files for the same period (17.5 million gallons). The Stellman team's data include an additional 1.6 million gallons in records covering the period before 1965 and the use of other agents.

EVALUATION OF THE INFRASTRUCTURE OF THE STELLMAN TEAM'S MODEL

In evaluating the infrastructure of the Stellman team's model, the issues of principal concern to the committee included the general completeness of the data, the completeness of data on herbicide spraying conducted separately from Ranch Hand flights, the potential for errors in the location of spraying arising from errors or imprecision in UTM coordinates or from the representation of flight paths as straight lines, and the appropriateness of assumptions about the extent of the area considered exposed to herbicide by a given mission. The committee included in its considerations limitations of the model noted by the Stellman team (e.g., Stellman and Stellman, 2004) as well as concerns about aspects of the model that have been raised by others (e.g., Young and Newton, 2004; Young et al., 2004a,b; Ross and Ginevan, 2007; Young, 2007; Ginevan et al., 2008).

Completeness of Data

Efforts have been made since the early 1970s to compile information about herbicide use in Vietnam. Records from the Vietnam War are known to vary in their quality and completeness (Shaughnessy, 1991; Young et al., 2004a; Boylan, 2007). Much of the data on which the HEA-V HERBS file is based were originally recorded by field units and forwarded to the Chemical Operations Division of the central military command in Vietnam.

A 1971 audit of an early version of the Ranch Hand spraying data characterized the statistical quality of the data as good; but it found that 2 percent of the records had missing data, 6 percent had "serious" transcription or measurement errors, and 23 percent had errors in the length of the track sprayed (Heizer, 1971). An assessment of the Ranch Hand records by a National Academy of Sciences committee (NRC, 1974) concluded that the data as a whole were reliable despite inaccuracies in some records. That committee's comparisons of flight path coordinates from a sample of records with aerial photographs suggested good agreement for defoliation missions.

The Stellman team has described a substantial review of various types of original records as part of its 1998–2003 work to develop its GIS and exposure opportunity model (Stellman and Stellman, 2003). The work was done in consultation with the Army unit now known as the Joint Services Records Research Center (JSRRC). The Stellman team used information they collected to fill in missing data on spraying records and to identify and correct errors when possible. In comparisons between the compiled records on spray missions and separate archival records on 60 percent of Ranch Hand target areas, spray paths of related missions were found to generally fall within these identified target areas (Stellman et al., 2003b). Because the Air Force target data and the mission flight path database are independent of each other and generally corroborate each other, the Stellman team sees them as providing some validation of the spray location data (Stellman et al., 2003b).

The committee is persuaded that the Stellman team's HERBS database is as complete a record of herbicide spraying as currently exists. However, the data appear to be more complete for the Air Force Ranch Hand missions than for spraying conducted by other services or by other means, such as helicopter or ground spraying. Because formal reporting for Army helicopter spraying is described as having started in 1968 (U.S. Army, 1985), the records on helicopter spraying are presumed to be more complete for the 1968–1971 period than for earlier years. To the committee's knowledge, factors influencing the availability of non-Ranch Hand spraying records have not been identified in any systematic way; it is therefore not possible to judge whether the available data are relatively representative or whether they may under-represent spraying activities in certain areas or time periods. The IOM committee that oversaw the Stellman team's work for VA reached a similar conclusion (IOM, 2003).

Accuracy of Flight Path Data

The Stellman team notes (Stellman and Stellman, 2004) that flight paths are represented with straight-line segments but that this assumption may not always hold. Young and colleagues (2004a) point to DAARs for reports that aircraft may have adopted zigzag flight patterns in response to enemy fire. The straight-line assumption may also not hold when the flight path followed features such as a river or a highway, with variations of as much as a kilometer or more from recorded locations suggested (Young et al., 2004a). Anecdotal evidence suggests that aircraft crews navigated by a combination of visual orientation and maps that were precise to no better than 120–240 meters (Young et al., 2004a).

The committee heard concerns that the Stellman team's EOI calculations take into account an excessively wide area (up to 5 kilometers) on either side of a flight path (Ross and Ginevan, 2007; Ginevan et al., 2008). This issue is discussed again later in the chapter, but the committee notes here that considering the wider area when assessing exposure opportunity would seem to address, at least to some extent, the concern that true flight paths may have deviated from the straight lines used in the model. Missions flown with multiple aircraft also would have contributed to variation in the width of the area where herbicide was applied.

Accuracy in locating herbicide spraying is essential for effective assessment of exposure, but the concerns that have been raised do not appear to point to major misrepresentations of locations in the spraying database.

Other Issues

It has been noted that troops on the ground may have mistaken the frequent aerial spraying of insecticide (e.g., malathion) for herbicide spraying (Young et al., 2004a; Cecil and Young, 2008). Young and colleagues (2004a) point to reports that between 1966 and 1972 more than 3.5 million liters of malathion were sprayed over approximately 6 million hectares of South Vietnam and that by 1970 malathion was being sprayed at 9-day intervals. The committee did not attempt to determine whether records exist that document the flight paths of insecticide spray missions. If they do, it would be appropriate to consider adding that data to the Stellman team's GIS.

THE STELLMAN TEAM'S EXPOSURE OPPORTUNITY METRICS

As previously described, the Stellman team's model produces two exposure metrics that are based on proximity to herbicide spraying: hits and the EOI. The hits metric represents direct exposure, and the EOI incorporates consideration of indirect exposure from previous spraying.

The model uses a two-stage approach to calculate the exposure values. The first stage relies on the datasets that the committee has described as the infrastructure of the model. The data on the location and date of each spraying mission are used to calculate a hit and an EOI value for each individual cell in the GIS grid that falls within 5 kilometers of that mission's spray path. These geographically based exposure calculations are stored, along with essential information about the associated spray mission, as individual records for each cell exposed to spraying during that mission. The database containing all this information (Exposure_Master) contains approximately 1.45 million records and is an integral part of the HEA-V tool.

At the second stage, this geographic exposure database is used in combination with user-supplied information on the location histories of military units, individual military personnel, or other study subjects to calculate exposure scores for the period that the units or the individuals spent in Vietnam.

Direct Exposure

The hits metric is generated for four specific distances from a spray path: 0.5, 1, 2, and 5 kilometers. A cell that fell within 0.5 kilometer of a given mission's spray path would have a hit score of 1 for each of the four distance possibilities. A cell that fell more than 2 kilometers but less than 5 kilometers from the flight path would have a hit score of 1 for only the 5-kilometer option. When information on military units or personnel is submitted for analysis, a GIS cell's hit scores for a given date are assigned to each individual or unit whose location history puts them in that cell on that date. The hit scores for a given distance option can be summed across spray missions to generate a cumulative score for a specified time period. For example, an HEA-V analysis found that during March 1969, 72 of 278 (15 percent) companies in Army combat battalions in III Corps were within 0.5 kilometer of a spray path (Stellman and Stellman, 2003). Of these units, 27 had cumulative scores for that month ranging from 2 to 19 for hits within the 0.5-kilometer distance.

Indirect Exposure Opportunity

The EOI calculation for each mission includes three main components: the amount of herbicide sprayed, a GIS cell's distance from the spray path, and an herbicide decay rate (Stellman and Stellman, 2003). The amount of herbicide is used as a concentration factor. Exposure is treated as inversely proportional to distance from the flight path (referred to as a 1/D factor), with calculations restricted to cells that are within 5 kilometers of the spray path. Herbicide decay is represented by a first-order decay model, with a 30-day half-life specified for the calculations at the geographic level. Users are given the option to specify an alternative half-life when calculations are made for military units or personnel.

For any given date, then, the EOI for a GIS cell reflects the combined effects of these three factors for any spraying that occurred on that date, plus the appropriate residual effect of previous spraying that impinged on that cell. In principle, these cell-specific EOI scores are cumulative for units or individuals in a manner similar to that for the hits score.

EVALUATION OF THE STELLMAN TEAM'S EXPOSURE OPPORTUNITY METRICS

Much of the criticism of the model has focused on the exposure metrics, generally with the argument that the metrics are inaccurate because the model fails to take into account other factors that influence the exposure of troops. The committee agrees that a number of potentially important factors have not been included in the Stellman team's model, and that many of these have the potential to cause misclassification of exposure that, if non-differential with respect to disease, will often tend to bias results toward the null. In other words, if the error in measuring exposure does not depend on disease, then the ability to associate exposure and disease will be reduced.

The committee found, however, that several of the criticisms reflect expectations of the model that extend beyond the capabilities of a proximity-based exposure opportunity approach. For example, concerns that the model does not take into account the chemical properties of the herbicides or the herbicide contaminant TCDD would be warranted for consideration in a model that purported to approximate the ambient levels of dioxin or herbicides in which troops operated in Vietnam (level 3 in Figure 3-1). As designed, however, the model provides only for the rough exposure classification permitted by assessing proximity to spray paths (level 2). With that in mind, the committee offers its assessment of the exposure opportunity metrics, including consideration of several criticisms.

Direct Exposure

The hits metric is calculated for distances from a spray path that range from 0.5 to 5 kilometers (i.e., a maximum swath 10 kilometers wide). This offers users the opportunity to assess the effect of different assumptions about proximity to spraying. In principle, modifications to the HEA-V would make it possible to use smaller distance factors, but the 1.2-square-kilometer resolution of the GIS grid imposes a limit on the precision with which small distances can be represented.

The committee heard concern that the model allows for attribution of exposure over an area that is much larger than the swath of 0.08–0.1 kilometer for a single C-123 fixed-wing aircraft (Ross and Ginevan, 2007; Ginevan et al., 2008). The area is also larger than the area that would be affected by spray drift as estimated from primary drift models (Ross and Ginevan, 2007) or that was affected in Air Force test flights (Young et al., 2004b). It was noted that even though spray missions typically involved multiple aircraft, the 80 percent that were flown with four or fewer planes would have generally have had a swath of no more than about 0.5 kilometer.

However, there is support for use of distances much greater than the nominal width of a plane's spray swath for an exposure opportunity metric. A 1969 report on herbicide use in South Vietnam included calculations that, under unfavorable but acceptable operating conditions, spray drift damage to broadleaf crops could occur at distances up to 2 kilometers (Darrow et al., 1969). The report also noted that unintended crop damage occurred on defoliation missions because of malfunctions of the spray equipment. An Army field manual on the use of herbicides indicated that crops should be safe from drift at a distance of 7 kilometers from spraying conducted with the equipment typically used on the C-123 Ranch Hand aircraft at the recommended altitude (150 feet) and close to the maximum acceptable ground wind speed (8 knots) (Department of the Army, 1971). Spray drift appeared evident in aerial photographs reviewed for a National Academy of Sciences study of the effects of herbicides in Vietnam (NRC, 1974). Whereas many spray swaths were reflected in bands with clearly defined boundaries, others showed a diffuse edge indicative of drift.

Indirect Exposure Opportunity

Concerns have been raised about some of the components of the EOI calculation: the herbicide decay rate, distance from the spray path as an exposure modifier, and the amount of herbicide sprayed. The decay rate is currently modifiable within the user interface of the software; therefore researchers who can support other half-life choices are free to use them for calculating the EOI. The model represents the effect on exposure of increasing distance from the spray path with an inverse distance (1/D) factor, which cannot be modified in the software's user interface. It would be useful if this were a changeable function in the software so that a researcher who could justify other drop-off rates could use them to calculate the EOI. An alternative to a simple drop-off rate in the EOI model would be to expand the EOI estimation to incorporate more advanced spray drift models (e.g., AgDRIFT®). This potential expansion of the model is discussed later in the chapter. The committee also noted that expanding the model to consider secondary drift might be useful in further addressing the effects of distance on exposure.

Another component of the Stellman team's EOI model is the amount of herbicide sprayed during a mission (gallonage), which is used to weight the EOI. Because herbicides were sprayed at a relatively constant rate over the flight path, herbicide gallonage is an indirect way to account for multi-plane missions along a single flight path. Since the HEA-V databases contain information for most fixed-wing missions on gallonage and the number of planes flying together, the model might benefit from incorporation of a better representation of the implicit width of the flight path. As noted previously, the Stellman team has explored methods to do this but has not incorporated this element into the current version of the HEA-V (Stellman, 2007). Given the availability of the data on gallonage and numbers of planes, other users of the model might be able to consider means of incorporating flight path width into EOI calculations.

Troop Presence

Although official policies have been described as ensuring that Ranch Hand spray targets were kept clear of U.S. troops during spray missions (Young et al., 2004a), the committee did not find that to be sufficient evidence that troops would not have been close to spray missions. In fact, GAO (1979) compared location data for Marine Corps infantry battalions for 1966 through 1969 with the location of Ranch Hand flights. Of 218,000 marines who served during that period, 5,900 were estimated to have been within 0.5 kilometer of a spray path on the day of the spraying, and 17,400 were within 2.5 kilometers. To the extent that documentation of troop locations near spraying exists, it must be taken as the best available evidence.

Proximity to Perimeter Spraying

As noted, the model calculates direct hits for a series of distances of from 0.5 to 5.0 kilometers from a fixed-wing flight path or the location of helicopter or ground spraying. It is possible, however, that drift from ground or helicopter spraying operations would have been less than that for spraying by fixed-wing aircraft, resulting in less exposure at a distance but more exposure near the spray path. Those operations may have been substantial contributors to exposure opportunity for at least some types of military units and their personnel.

In the analyses done in conjunction with the planning for the CDC Agent Orange Study, most hits (i.e., presence within 2 kilometers of spraying within the previous 6 days) were found to be from helicopter and ground spraying, including perimeter spraying of fire bases (CDC, 1989). Likewise, when the Stellman team's GIS was used to investigate exposures of stable units in March 1969, it was found that 2 percent (36) of the 1,982 unit locations had hits within 0.5 kilometer from fixed-wing spraying, and 7 percent (141) had hits within 0.5 kilometer from helicopter and ground spraying (Stellman and Stellman, 2003). If the hit zone is widened to 5 kilometers, 10 percent of the locations had hits from fixed-wing spraying and 18 percent had hits from perimeter spraying during the month.

For the subset of operations that involve spraying the perimeter of a base, it may be possible to match the base coordinates with the coordinates in the HERBS files to assign "hits" to bases during that spray event.

Spray Penetration

It was suggested to the committee that little of the herbicide sprayed actually made it to the forest floor where ground troops could be exposed (Ross and Ginevan, 2007; Young, 2007). Some of the herbicide applied would be absorbed into the waxy layer of the plants and most of this absorbed herbicide would undergo photodegradation by ultraviolet radiation in a few hours. TCDD has been shown to have a photodegradation half-life of 6 to 10 hours under some conditions (Young et al., 2004b).

A report describes experiments by the U.S. Department of Agriculture in Puerto Rico and Texas finding that on average 21 percent of the spray penetrated the upper canopy and 6 percent penetrated to ground level (Young et al., 2004a). Young and colleagues (2004a) also note that a "leaf area index" for the Vietnamese jungle predicts that only 1 percent to 6 percent of an aerial spray would have reached the lowest levels. However, this does not appear to account for spraying in areas where the amount of protective foliage was more sparse or may have diminished over time as a result of previous spraying.

As noted, calculations using the Stellman team's HERBS database show that approximately 95 percent of the herbicide known to have been used in Vietnam was applied via fixed-wing aircraft. The remainder was dispersed via helicopters or ground-based spraying. The assumptions made about the proportion of herbicide reaching the ground from fixed-wing spraying in comparison with other application methods would be important in judging the contribution of each source to a more refined estimate of exposure opportunity. This sort of refinement would require more detailed data regarding factors such as canopy cover and remaining canopy for previously sprayed areas, which would move beyond the proximity-based approach adopted by the Stellman team. The committee also notes that while such adjustments offer the potential to provide more local detail to measures of exposure opportunity, the geographic size of the grid cells underlying the GIS presents a practical limit to the ultimate spatial resolution of any such adjustments.

TCDD Exposure

In its current form, the Stellman team's model does not offer means of generating exposure scores linked specifically to TCDD. Although it is possible to calculate scores specifically for exposure to Agent Orange and the other herbicides that contained 2,4,5-T, the level of TCDD contamination in these herbicides varied over time and by several orders of magnitude (from less than 0.05 ppm to 50 ppm; IOM, 1994). Because the model incorporates no adjustments for varying levels of TCDD, the potential exists for misclassification in estimates of exposure to TCDD. This implies that the model will generally be better suited for examining exposure to herbicides than for examining exposure to TCDD.

Does the EOI Produce a Range of Potential Exposure Values?

For exposure measures to be useful in epidemiology, they must show a range of exposure in the population under study. To investigate the range of potential exposures among Vietnam veterans, the Stellman team identified 1,957 "stable" Army units in Vietnam in June 1969 and the 2,095 cells in the GIS grid that these units occupied during that month (Stellman et al., 2003b). Of the 2,095 occupied cells, 56 percent of the locations had been sprayed and were occupied by 1,045 units. Personnel counts could be estimated for 815 of these units and totaled 142,583 soldiers. The resulting distribution of EOI scores for these soldiers was lognormal and spanned several orders of magnitude (see Figure 3-2).

However, unpublished calculations provided to the committee (now published as Ginevan et al., 2008) gave results showing that in some instances the EOI scores of locations directly under a flight path and locations as much as 4 kilometers away from the flight path are not significantly different. Although the implications of these differences are unclear, the

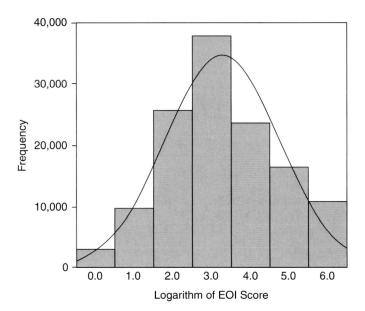

FIGURE 3-2 Frequency distribution of the logarithm of the non-zero EOI scores for 142,583 soldiers in 815 units designated as "stable" or "stable with mobile elements," June 1969.
SOURCE: Stellman et al., 2003b. Reproduced with permission from *Environmental Health Perspectives*.

committee urges, as discussed below, that more sensitivity testing be done to gain a better understanding of the dynamics of the model.

The committee also emphasizes that the EOI data do not describe the magnitude of exposure in units that can be used to make comparisons with exposures measured in other populations. Because EOI is a proximity measure that does not account for fate and transport, personal activity patterns, or biological uptake characteristics, it seems unlikely that the EOI will be proportional to exposure. Instead, the measure is more likely to be a reasonable means of ranking potential exposure.

Comparison of the Hit Score and EOI

The committee sees strengths and weaknesses in both of the Stellman team's proximity-based exposure opportunity measures. The hit score has the virtue of being very simple. However, when used as an exposure surrogate, it implicitly makes two assumptions that are likely to cause exposure misclassification: (1) residual herbicide does not contribute to future exposure (i.e., as if it has a short half-life in the environment), and (2) distribution of herbicide is uniform within the assigned radius (i.e., ignoring drop-off with distance from the flight path). The EOI takes into account both the presence of residual herbicide (via the decay rate) and distance, but it does this in ways that may not be accurate. For example, it was not clear to the committee that the current procedure of integration of the 1/D function along the flight path is the best approach. Both hits and the EOI have merits, but both are likely to cause some level of exposure misclassification.

Sensitivity Analyses Needed

Given the nature of the proximity-based exposure opportunity measures and the associated assumptions regarding decreases in herbicide concentration with distance and time, the committee stresses the importance of quantitative assessments of the sensitivity of these measures to the model assumptions. Such assessments are often based on recording the amount of variation in model outputs resulting from systematic variation of model inputs (e.g., distance from the flight path in the "hits" approach, or the rate of distance-decay in the EOI). In the case of the HEA-V software, general sensitivity analyses could involve summaries of exposure opportunity scores associated with particular units or individuals, or, more broadly, involve local summaries (ranges, distributions, or percentiles) of exposure opportunity scores mapped for each of a number of grid cells. An initial effort in this direction is reflected by the Stellman team's evaluation of the impact of small shifts in the coordinates, which suggested minimal impact on exposure assignment (Stellman and Stellman, 2003). It is important to note that such analyses can be conducted even in the absence of "gold standard" exposure measures. They provide information on the stability of the proposed measures under uncertainty around model inputs and assumptions, and they provide important context for any epidemiologic study in which the measures are used.

Additional directions researchers might pursue include more detailed statistical modeling of data uncertainties, including models of measurement error. However, in the absence of a gold standard by which to evaluate error, researchers face a challenge. If they are able to estimate the likely distribution of errors in the study population and thus quantify the range in uncertainty, this should be taken into account in sensitivity analyses and power calculations.

POTENTIAL FOR CORROBORATION OF EXPOSURE MEASURES

In large retrospective occupational or environmental studies, it is often impossible to obtain detailed exposure information for all subjects. When a surrogate measure on the exposure assessment hierarchy (see Figure 3-1) is used instead, it is then desirable to compare the surrogate with other exposure indicators. In the case of the Stellman team's exposure opportunity model, correlation of the EOI with variations in TCDD levels in independent environmental data or in tissue samples could theoretically increase confidence in the model's measures of exposure opportunity for the herbicides that contained the TCDD contaminant. Unfortunately, neither approach appears likely to be sufficiently informative to be worthwhile.

Utility of TCDD Measurements in Soil, Water, and Sediments

It is estimated that the use of herbicides in Vietnam resulted in the deposition of between 170 and 680 kilograms of TCCD over the southern part of the country (Dwernychuk et al., 2002). Although TCDD persists in the environment, the committee sees little opportunity to use information on its current levels to provide more than broad qualitative support for the Stellman team's model.

TCDD is part of a family of polychlorinated dibenzo-p-dioxins (PCDDs) which are often found together. The mix of PCDDs varies depending on their source. They are byproducts of low-temperature combustion processes, such as the open burning of waste material, and they are also generated during the production or use of some chlorinated chemical products, including phenoxy herbicides such as Agent Orange (ATSDR, 1998). TCDD was present as a PCDD contaminant of special concern in the 2,4,5-T herbicide used in Agent Orange and in some of the other military herbicides used in Vietnam, but it is not prominent in PCDDs generated by combustion.

TCDD and related compounds have very low water solubility and are lipophilic. Following aerial spraying, waste incineration, or other atmospheric releases, the compounds may be deposited on plants, on soil, and in bodies of water and their sediments. They can also enter water and sediments from such sources as effluent discharge and soil runoff. Although TCDD can be degraded by sunlight, it is otherwise highly persistent in the environment and can accumulate in the fatty tissue of some fish and mammals. Studies carried out at Eglin Air Force Base in Florida indicated that even though 99 percent of the TCDD applied was photodegraded, TCDD was still detectable in test plots several years after application (Young and Newton, 2004). The half-life of TCDD has been estimated at 9–15 years in surface soil and 25–100 years in subsurface soil (Paustenbach et al., 1992). In sediments, TCDD has been found to persist over decades (Bopp et al., 1991).

An investigation in one area of Vietnam found that TCDD levels were somewhat elevated in soil samples from locations where aerial spraying had occurred 30 years earlier (Dwernychuk et al., 2002). The same investigation also found that soil samples from Special Forces bases in the area had significantly higher concentrations of TCDD than the soil samples collected from flight paths. The higher levels in the base areas were attributed to herbicide spillage and disposal. A separate analysis of soil and sediment from areas at and around the site of the Da Nang Airbase, which was a base used for Operation Ranch Hand missions, found very high levels of TCDD (365,000 ppt) in soil samples from specific sites where herbicides had been stored or airplanes' spray tanks had been loaded (Hatfield Consultants and Office of the National Steering Committee 33, MNRE, 2007).

Because of the persistence of TCDD and other PCDDs, samples of undisturbed soil or sediment can provide a historical record of their deposition (e.g., Czuczwa and Hites, 1984, 1986; Baker and Hites, 2000). Comparisons of TCDD and PCDD levels found in areas that were sprayed and areas that were not may offer some qualitative insight into past exposure sources. However, several factors hinder the use of data on current TCDD concentrations to validate the Stellman team's model. With sediment cores from a lake or delta, the historical profile of the total levels of TCDD deposited over the watershed does not adequately indicate localized variations in soil deposition. In addition, the precision with which TCDD deposition in sediments can be dated is limited and may be no better than 2 to 5 years (e.g., Frignani et al., 2004). Therefore sediment analysis could only be used to validate the estimates of exposure opportunity generated by the Stellman team's model on very broad geographic and temporal scales.

With soil analysis, the range of 9 to 15 years for the estimated half-life of TCDD in surface soil and the use of herbicides extending over a 10-year period mean that present-day TCDD levels may reflect levels that were anywhere from 3.4 to 15 times higher during the war. There are also likely to have been other sources of TCDD and PCDD deposition over the more than 45 years since herbicide spraying began, including contributions from open burning of waste during and after the war, burning of materials containing polychlorinated biphenyls, and long-range atmospheric transport of TCDD and PCDDs. As a result, it may be difficult to isolate the contributions of TCDD from war-era herbicides except in areas where they were extensively used.

For the herbicides themselves that were used in Vietnam, virtually no opportunity exists to test for residues. The principal components of Agent Orange, the military herbicide used most extensively, were 2,4-D and 2,4,5-T in various formulations. Unlike TCDD, these compounds are fairly water soluble and not persistent. For example, 2,4-T has a half-life in soil of approximately 6 days and in aerobic aquatic environments of 15 days (EPA, 2005). Similarly, malathion, which was sprayed to control mosquitoes and potentially confused with herbicide spraying, has a half life of 11 days or less in soil and up to 2 weeks in an aerobic aquatic environment (EPA, 2006). As a result, no major accumulation of these compounds in soil and sediment is likely.

Utility of Serum and Adipose TCDD Measurements

In humans, an initial rapid rate of elimination of TCDD is followed by a slower rate that results in an estimated half-life of 7–10 years (e.g., Michalek et al., 2002). As it has been more than 35 years since any U.S. military personnel were exposed to TCDD in Vietnam, studies conducted now may not be able to reliably distinguish TCDD exposure in Vietnam from background exposure in the United States from other sources (e.g., combustion or food). The IOM committee that oversaw the Stellman team's work for VA reached a similar conclusion (IOM, 2003). Some previous studies have explored the correlation between measures of exposure and TCDD levels in tissue samples. These studies have used various approaches to exposure measurement and have had varying results.

CDC Study

In 1987, CDC (1988, 1989) measured TCDD levels in serum samples from 646 enlisted Vietnam veterans with a pay grade between E1 and E5 and only one tour of duty in Vietnam (average 320 days) who served in one of five combat battalions in III Corps during 1967–1968. Comparison samples were drawn from 97 U.S. Army veterans of the same era who did not serve in Vietnam (CDC, 1988). The Vietnam veterans were selected to represent low, medium, and high categories of exposure, which were defined on the basis of the number of hits. (As described above, a hit was defined as a person's company being located within 2 kilometers of a recorded Agent Orange spraying mission within 6 days after the spraying.) Subjects in the high exposure category had five or more hits. Fifty-four percent of the Vietnam veterans enrolled in the study had at least one hit, and 30 percent had five or more. The analysis used this exposure measure as well as two others, all of which were based on proximity in space and time to Agent Orange spraying, as the Stellman team's measures are.

Although a range of TCDD levels was found in this study, the serum levels of those who served in Vietnam, which ranged from non-detectable levels to 45 ng/g lipid, were not significantly different from the levels among veterans with no Vietnam service (range: non-detectable levels to 25 ng/g lipid) (CDC, 1988). Only 4 percent of the Vietnam veterans had TCDD levels above 8 ng/g lipid. There was also no significant trend in serum TCDD levels by exposure score category. The lack of relationship between serum TCDD levels and exposure scores was an important factor in the cancellation of the larger CDC study of the long-term health effects of exposure to Agent Orange (CDC, 1989).

There are several reasons why the CDC study may have failed to detect a difference in TCDD serum concentrations between the veterans who served in Vietnam and those who did not. The TCDD concentrations in Agent Orange used during the exposure period studied may have been relatively low. Contamination levels could vary by production run and manufacturer and were found to range from 0.05 to 50 ppm, averaging 1.98 and 2.99 in two sets of samples (NRC, 1974; Young et al., 1978).

It is also possible that the study selection criterion requiring a single tour of duty may have undersampled subjects with high exposure opportunity, limiting the power of the study to detect differences. Only 30 percent of the Vietnam veterans tested had hit scores of 5 or greater (i.e., being in locations within 2 kilometers of spraying that had occurred in the previous 6 days five or more times).

Differences in pharmacokinetics between veterans due to differences in metabolism, body composition, or weight change, could have influenced the rate at which TCDD was eliminated. Furthermore, the pharmacokinetics of TCDD is more complicated than the simple first-order models assumed in the CDC study as the basis for power calculations (e.g., Michalek et al., 2002; Emond et al., 2005). However, elevated serum and adipose tissue levels of TCDD have been used elsewhere to document higher exposure (e.g., Flesch-Janys et al., 1998; Michalek et al., 2002).

Another possibility is that most American military personnel who served in Vietnam did not have high TCDD exposure. The range of exposure opportunity scores seen for most Vietnam veterans may not represent significant elevations in TCDD exposure. The lack of correlation between exposure score and TCDD serum levels could also mean that the exposure score is a poor surrogate for TCDD exposure.

Residents of Vietnam

Comparisons have also been made between TCDD levels and EOIs for two groups of Vietnamese (Verger et al., 1994; Kramarova et al., 1998; Stellman and Stellman, 2003). In one comparison, adipose tissue samples from 25 participants in a cancer case-control study conducted in Ho Chi Minh City were analyzed for TCDD and other PCDDs and PCDFs (Stellman and Stellman, 2003). These subjects were recruited in 1993–1997 for a study supervised by the International Agency for Research on Cancer (IARC). Of the analyzed samples (from a mix of cases and controls), 11 had detectable TCDD levels, ranging from 1.0 to 4.2 pg/g lipid. The Stellman team (Stellman and Stellman, 2003) computed EOI values for the study subjects on the basis of geocoded residential histories. Seven subjects had an EOI of zero; scores for the others ranged from 295 to 7.7×10^5. The Pearson correlation coefficient between the TCDD levels and the EOI (both log-transformed) was 0.23 and not significantly different from zero, but no sample had both a high TCDD level and a low EOI (Stellman and Stellman, 2003).

A second study examined 27 Vietnamese men admitted for abdominal surgery in Ho Chi Minh City in 1989; all patients were born before 1953 (Verger et al., 1994). TCDD concentrations in adipose tissue samples (range: non-detectable levels to 49.6 pg/g lipid) were compared with EOI scores (range: 0 to 9,868) computed based on residential history and an earlier version of the Stellman team's model. The Spearman correlation coefficient for all samples was 0.32, $p = 0.10$ (with log transformation: Pearson $r = 0.36$, $p = 0.07$). Restricting the analysis to the 22 subjects with non-zero EOIs increased the correlation (Spearman = 0.44, $p = 0.04$; Pearson = 0.50, $p = 0.02$) (Verger et al., 1994; Stellman and Stellman, 2003).

The committee sees the data on Vietnamese residents as providing weak evidence that the EOI can serve as a predictor of TCDD concentrations in people. It is unclear whether these results can be generalized to U.S. veterans because the Vietnamese study subjects could have been exposed to TCDD for long periods of time, including extended exposure via the food chain, a route less likely for American military personnel.

TESTING AND REFINING THE STELLMAN TEAM'S MODEL

The Stellman team's model for herbicide exposure in Vietnam counts direct exposure events and also produces a quantitative representation of indirect exposure that takes account of the quantity of herbicide sprayed, the distance from the spray path, and, by using an environmental decay factor for the herbicides, the time since spraying. The committee notes first that the exposure assessment model and metrics developed by the Stellman team are one approach but not necessarily the only approach that might be followed for a proximity-based assessment of exposure opportunity. Other approaches might be explored, possibly without requiring collection of additional data.

There are also several possible expansions of the model and the GIS databases, each of which has advantages and disadvantages. For example, the Stellman team (Stellman et al., 2003b) has described developing other geocoded databases that might be used to refine exposure estimates. Examples of these databases include locations of inhabited places during the period of the Vietnam War, roadways and other constructed features, locations of military sites, and soil types. Only the database on soil types was available to the committee for examination.

Aerial spray drift dispersion models might also be useful. For example, the AgDRIFT (Teske et al., 2002) and AGDISP models (Bilanin et al., 1989) use inputs such as the type of aircraft and spray nozzle, characteristics of the spray material, spraying height, swath width, wind speed and direction, and temperature to estimate the percentage of the spray that deposits at various distances from the flight path. For application to spraying in Vietnam, inputs such as weather conditions are likely to be available from the DAARs, but they would have varied relatively little if official operating procedures were followed. Those procedures specified that spraying flights take place in clear weather, with wind speeds of no more than 10 miles per hour, and that herbicide be dispensed at an altitude of 150 feet at a constant delivery rate of 3 gallons/acre (MACV, 1969; Stellman and Stellman, 2003; Young et al., 2004a).

Other factors such as the types of vegetation, characteristics of the initial and remaining canopy, and meteorological parameters that could affect the ground-level deposition, photodegradation rate, and the availability of herbicide in the topsoil could also be incorporated into a more detailed exposure model that might use the Stellman team's EOI or the spraying location data in the GIS as a starting point. Consideration of secondary drift (e.g., through evaporation from treated plant materials or transport of aerosolized particles) might further improve estimation of exposure. However, the committee is not aware of any currently existing secondary drift models that could be directly applied. Rather, such models would need to be developed.

Although use of spray drift models or incorporation of other factors could potentially result in improved quantification of herbicide deposition, it is unclear whether they would result in changes in the relative ranking of

ASSESSMENT OF THE MODEL 59

exposures among military personnel or units. It is also unclear how much of the historical data needed to use these more advanced spray deposition models would be available in the military records.

No "gold standard" exists for use in testing the accuracy of retrospectively estimated exposure of veterans to herbicides in Vietnam using the Stellman team's hits or EOI score, alternative simple proximity-based measures (e.g., incorporating other distance functions), or approaches that use the Stellman team's infrastructure as a foundation for more elaborate fate and transport modeling (e.g., primary and secondary drift). Thus the committee sees it as essential that sensitivity analyses be done to compare various approaches to estimating exposure. The exposure measures they produce should be compared with each other to see how assigned exposures are changed, particularly rank orderings. The impact of assumptions (e.g., distance functions, decay rates) should be examined in the same way.

CONCLUSIONS

Based on its review of the Stellman team's herbicide exposure assessment model, the committee reached several conclusions.

1. Using a surrogate of exposure that is based on individuals' or military units' proximity in space and time to herbicide spray paths is a reasonable exposure assessment strategy. This approach is a clear improvement over the cruder measures of exposure or opportunity for exposure, such as those based on service in Vietnam, that have been used in some past studies of the potential effects of herbicide exposure on the health of Vietnam veterans. Such proximity-based surrogates are similar to exposure measures commonly used in occupational health studies (e.g., job title) and in environmental studies of proximity to sources of exposure.

2. The Stellman team's databases and GIS provide a useful basis for estimating proximity-based surrogates of exposure to herbicides in Vietnam. Because of the availability of relatively more complete data on spraying by fixed-wing aircraft, the model is currently better suited to examining proximity to that type of spraying than to spraying from ground equipment or helicopters. The uncertainty about the completeness of the data on helicopter and ground spraying should be taken into consideration, especially when studying stable units, which may have had limited exposure to fixed-wing spraying.

3. The Stellman team's hits and EOI scores have value in that they move further along the exposure assessment hierarchy than exposure assessment based only on presence in Vietnam. However, the methods by which the hits and EOI scores are calculated have the potential for significant exposure misclassification, and so these metrics must be used with caution.

Other proximity-based approaches with the potential for estimating exposure scores more accurately should be explored. Moving from exposure metrics based on spray and troop location data to more accurate exposure and dose metrics would require the incorporation of additional data, such as herbicide fate and transport, individual behavior, and pharmacokinetics.

4. Fate and transport processes not incorporated into the current version of the Stellman team's model (e.g., width of the spray swath, concentration of contaminants, primary and secondary drift, soil conditions, initial and remaining canopy, and photodegradation) will affect estimates of exposure to herbicides and their contaminants. Incorporating these phenomena into an exposure model could possibly reduce exposure misclassification but would require additional data that may or may not be available. However, the relatively coarse resolution of the military UTM system used in military records and the Stellman team's GIS grid map of Vietnam may limit, to some extent, the benefits of adding fine-scale fate and transport modeling.

5. Regardless of the exposure model used, sensitivity analyses are necessary to determine the impact of model assumptions regarding decreases in herbicide concentration with distance and time on the exposure assignments generated. Such studies provide important information on the stability of the proposed exposure opportunity measures.

6. Given the significant uncertainties about the levels of TCDD contamination over time and from different lots of the herbicides used in Vietnam, proximity-based exposure models may be better suited to studies of the health effects of herbicides in general rather than TCDD specifically.

7. It is not feasible to validate the exposure scores produced by the Stellman team's model, or any other proximity-based model, by comparisons with biomarker or soil samples because of the passage of time and the unavailability of archived environmental or biological samples.

RESEARCH OPPORTUNITIES

From its review of the Stellman team's model, the committee identified two areas where it urges further investigation.

1. Efforts should be made to improve and refine the Stellman team's model by exploring alternative formulations of the proximity-based exposure metrics and by incorporating alternative or additional model parameters that account for more aspects of herbicide fate and transport in the environment. Further development of the model will require an assessment of the additional data needed and of the availability of these data.

2. The sensitivity of the Stellman team's model's results to changes in parameter values should be assessed systematically. The committee specifi-

cally urges attention to effects of potential inaccuracies in the data on the location of herbicide application or troop presence. It is also important to investigate, especially with any attempt to add refinements to the existing model, the effect of assumptions on factors such as spray swath, the concentration of the TCDD contamination, primary and secondary drift, soil conditions, initial and remaining canopy, and photodegradation of sprayed herbicide. Although the committee concluded, based on the information it reviewed, that direct validation of the accuracy of exposure assignment is not feasible, it encourages efforts to quantify the degree of accuracy and incorporate those estimates into the sensitivity analysis.

REFERENCES

ATSDR (Agency for Toxic Substances and Disease Registry). 1998. *Toxicological profile for chlorinated dibenzo-p-dioxins*. Atlanta, GA: U.S. Department of Health and Human Services.

Baker, J. I., and R. A. Hites. 2000. Siskiwit Lake revisited: Time trend of polychlorinated dibenzo-*p*-dioxins and dibenzofuran deposited at Isle Royale, Michigan. *Environmental Science and Technology* 34:2887–2891.

Bertazzi, P. A., I. Bernucci, G. Brambilla, D. Consonni, and A. C. Pesatori. 1998. The Seveso studies on early and long-term effects of dioxin exposure: A review. *Environmental Health Perspectives* 106(S2):625–633.

Bertazzi, P. A., D. Consonni, S. Bachetti, M. Rubagotti, A. Baccarelli, C. Zocchetti, and A. C. Pesatori. 2001. Health effects of dioxin exposure: A 20-year mortality study. *American Journal of Epidemiology* 153(11):1031–1044.

Bilanin, A. J., M. E. Teske, J. W. Barry, and R. B. Ekblad. 1989. AGDISP: The aircraft spray dispersion model, code development and experimental validation. *Transactions of the American Society of Agricultural Engineers* 32:327–334.

Bopp, R. F., M. L. Gross, H. Tong, H. J. Simpson, S. J. Monson, B. L. Deck, and F. C. Moser. 1991. A major incident of dioxin contamination: Sediments of New Jersey estuaries. *Environmental Science and Technology* 25(5):951–956.

Boylan, R. 2007. *Accessing military unit records at the College Park Archives*. Oral presentation to the IOM Committee on Making Best Use of the Agent Orange Reconstruction Model, Meeting 2, April 30–May 1, Washington, DC.

Caramaschi, F., G. del Corno, C. Favaretti, S. E. Giambelluca, E. Montesarchio, and G. M. Fara. 1981. Chloracne following environmental contamination by TCDD in Seveso, Italy. *International Journal of Epidemiology* 10(2):135–143.

CDC (Centers for Disease Control and Prevention). 1988. Serum 2,3,7,8-tetrachlorodibenzo-*p*-dioxin levels in U.S. Army Vietnam-era veterans. *Journal of the American Medical Association* 260(9):1249–1254.

CDC. 1989. *Comparison of serum levels of 2,3,7,8-tetrachlorodibenzo-p-dioxin with indirect estimates of Agent Orange exposure among Vietnam veterans: Final report*. Atlanta, GA: Agent Orange Projects, Center for Environmental Health and Injury Control.

Cecil, P. F., Sr., and A. L. Young. 2008. Operation FLYSWATTER: A war within a war. *Environmental Science and Pollution Research* 15(1):3–7.

Curwin, B. D., M. J. Hein, W. T. Sanderson, M. G. Nishioka, S. J. Reynolds, E. M. Ward, and M. C. Alavanja. 2005. Pesticide contamination inside farm and nonfarm homes. *Journal of Occupational and Environmental Hygiene* 2(7):357–367.

Czuczwa, J. M., and R. A. Hites. 1984. Environmental fate of combustion-generated polychlorinated dioxins and furans. *Environmental Science and Technology* 18(6):444–450.

Czuczwa, J. M., and R. A. Hites. 1986. Airborne dioxins and dibenzofurans: Sources and fates. *Environmental Science and Technology* 20(2):195–200.

Darrow, R. A., K. R. Irish, and C E. Hinarik. 1969. *Herbicides used in Southeast Asia.* Technical Report SAOQ-TR-69-11078. Fort Detrick, MD: U.S. Army Plant Sciences Laboratories.

Department of the Army. 1971. *Tactical employment of herbicides.* Field Manual FM 3-3. Washington, DC: Department of the Army.

Dwernychuk, L. W., H. D. Cau, C. T. Hatfield, T. G. Boivin, T. M. Hung, P. T. Dung, and N. D. Thai. 2002. Dioxin reservoirs in southern Viet Nam: A legacy of Agent Orange. *Chemosphere* 47:117–137.

Emond, E., J. E. Michalek, L. S. Birnbaum, and M. J. DeVito. 2005. Comparison of the use of a physiology based pharmacokinetic model and a classical pharmacokinetic model for dioxin exposure assessments. *Environmental Health Perspectives* 113(12):1666–1674.

EPA (Environmental Protection Agency). 2005. *2,4-D RED facts.* EPA-738F-05-002. http://www.epa.gov/oppsrrd1/REDs/factsheets/24d_fs.htm (accessed December 4, 2007).

EPA. 2006. *Reregistration eligibility decision (RED) for malathion.* EPA 738-R-06-030. http://www.epa.gov/pesticides/reregistration/REDs/malathion_red.pdf (accessed December 4, 2007).

Eskenazi, B., P. Mocarelli, M. Warner, L. Needham, D. G. Patterson, Jr., S. Samuels, W. Turner, P. M. Gerthoux, and P. Brambilla. 2004. Relationship of serum TCDD concentrations and age at exposure of female residents of Seveso, Italy. *Environmental Health Perspectives* 112(1):22–27.

Flesch-Janys, D., K. Steindorf, P. Gurn, and H. Becher. 1998. Estimation of the cumulated exposure to polychlorinated dibenzo-*p*-dioxins/furans and standardized mortality ratio analysis of cancer mortality by dose in an occupationally exposed cohort. *Environmental Health Perspectives* 106(S2):655–662.

Frignani, M., R. Piazza, L. G. Bellucci, C. N. Huu, R. Zangrando, S. Albertazzi, and I. Moret. 2004. Polychlorinated biphenyls in sediments of the Tam Giang-Cau Hai Lagoon (Central Vietnam): First results. *Organohalogen Compounds* 66:3657–3663.

GAO (General Accounting Office). 1979. *U.S. ground troops in South Vietnam were in areas sprayed with Herbicide Orange.* FPCD-80-23. Washington, DC: U.S. Government Printing Office.

Ginevan, M. E., J. H. Ross, and D. K. Watkins. 2008. Assessing exposure to allied ground troops in the Vietnam War: A comparison of AgDRIFT and exposure opportunity index models. *Journal of Exposure Science and Environmental Epidemiology* advance online publication, March 12 (DOI:10.1038/sj.jes.2008.12).

Hatfield Consultants and Office of the National Steering Committee 33, MNRE (Ministry of Natural Resources and Environment, Vietnam). 2007. *Assessment of dioxin contamination in the environment and human population in the vicinity of Da Nang Airbase, Viet Nam: Final report.* West Vancouver, British Columbia, Canada.

HEA-V (Herbicide Exposure Assessment–Vietnam). 2003. *CD-ROM, version 1.0.2. Software and accompanying electronic documentation.* New York: Columbia University.

Heizer, J. R. 1971. *Data quality analysis of the HERB 01 data file.* MITRE Technical Report, MTR-5105. Prepared for the Defense Communications Agency. McLean, VA: MITRE.

IOM (Institute of Medicine). 1994. *Veterans and Agent Orange: Health effects of herbicides used in Vietnam.* Washington, DC: National Academy Press.

IOM. 2003. *Characterizing exposure of veterans to Agent Orange and other herbicides used in Vietnam: Interim findings and recommendations.* Washington, DC: The National Academies Press.

Koch, D., C. Lu, J. Fisker-Andersen, L. Jolley, and R. A. Fenske. 2002. Temporal association of children's pesticide exposure and agricultural spraying: Report of a longitudinal biological monitoring study. *Environmental Health Perspectives* 110(8):829–833.

Kramarova, E., M. Kogevinas, C. T. Anh, H. D. Cau, L. C. Dai, S. D. Stellman, and D. M. Parkin. 1998. Exposure to Agent Orange and occurrence of soft-tissue sarcomas or non-Hodgkin lymphomas: An ongoing study in Vietnam. *Environmental Health Perspectives* 106(Suppl 2):671–678.

Lu, C., R. A. Fenske, N. Simcox, and D. Kalman. 2000. Pesticide exposure of children in an agricultural community: Evidence of household proximity to farmland and take home exposure pathways. *Environmental Research* 84(3):290–302.

MACV (Military Assistance Command, Vietnam). 1969. *Military operations: Herbicide operations*. Directive 525-1. Springfield, VA: National Technical Information Service.

Michalek, J. E., J. L. Pirkle, L. L. Needham, D. G. Patterson, Jr., S. P. Caudill, R. C. Tripathi, and P. Mocarelli. 2002. Pharmacokinetics of 2,3,7,8-tetrachlorodibenzo-*p*-dioxin in Seveso adults and veterans of operation Ranch Hand. *Journal of Exposure Analysis and Environmental Epidemiology* 12:44–53.

NRC (National Research Council). 1974. *The effects of herbicides in Vietnam. Part A—Summary and conclusions*. Washington, DC: National Academy of Sciences.

Paustenbach, D. J., R. J. Wenning, V. Lau, N. W. Harrington, D. K. Rennix, and A. H. Parsons. 1992. Recent developments on the hazards posed by 2,3,7,8-tetrachlorodibenzo-*p*-dioxin in soil: Implications for setting risk-based cleanup levels at residential and industrial sites. *Journal of Toxicology and Environmental Health* 36(2):103–149.

Ross, J. H., and M. E. Ginevan. 2007. *Points for the committee to consider when evaluating the Stellman model*. PowerPoint presentation to the IOM Committee on Making Best Use of the Agent Orange Exposure Reconstruction Model, Meeting 2, April 30–May 1, Washington, DC.

Shaughnessy, C. A. 1991. The Vietnam conflict: "America's best documented war"? *The History Teacher* 24(2):135–147.

Stanton, S. L. 1989. Area-scoring methodology for estimating Agent Orange exposure status of U.S. Army personnel in the Republic of Vietnam. In *Comparison of serum levels of 2,3,7,8-tetrachlorodibenzo-p-dioxin with indirect estimates of Agent Orange exposure among Vietnam veterans: Final report*, by Centers for Disease Control and Prevention. Atlanta, GA: Agent Orange Projects, Center for Environmental Health and Injury Control.

Stellman, J. M. 2007. *Responses to IOM 091407*. Unpublished document submitted to the IOM Committee on Making the Best Use of the Agent Orange Reconstruction Model, September 14.

Stellman, J. M., and S. D. Stellman. 2003. *Contractor's final report: Characterizing exposure of veterans to Agent Orange and other herbicides in Vietnam*. Submitted to the National Academy of Sciences, Institute of Medicine, in fulfillment of Subcontract VA-5124-98-0019, June 30, 2003.

Stellman, S. D., and J. M. Stellman. 2004. Exposure opportunity models for Agent Orange, dioxin, and other military herbicides used in Vietnam, 1961–1971. *Journal of Exposure Analysis and Environmental Epidemiology* 14(4):354–362.

Stellman, J. M., S. D. Stellman, R. Christian, T. Weber, and C. Tomasallo. 2003a. The extent and patterns of usage of Agent Orange and other herbicides in Vietnam. *Nature* 422(6933):681–687.

Stellman, J. M., S. D. Stellman, T. Weber, C. Tomasallo, A. B. Stellman, and R. Christian, Jr. 2003b. A geographic information system for characterizing exposure to Agent Orange and other herbicides in Vietnam. *Environmental Health Perspectives* 111(3):321–328.

Teske, M. E., S. L. Bird, D. M. Esterly, T. B. Curbishly, S. L. Ray, and S. G. Perry. 2002. AgDRIFT®: A model for estimating near-field spray drift from aerial applications. *Environmental Toxicology and Chemistry* 21(3):659–671.

U.S. Army. 1985. *Services HERBS Tape*. Report No. AD-A160 563. Washington, DC: U.S. Army and Joint Services Environmental Support Group.

Verger, P., S. Cordier, L. T. B. Thuy, D. Bard, L. C. Dai, P. H. Phiet, M. F. Gonnord, and L. Abenhaim. 1994. Correlation between dioxin levels in adipose tissue and estimated exposure to Agent Orange in South Vietnamese residents. *Environmental Research* 65:226–242.

Ward, M. H., J. Lubin, J. Giglierano, J. S. Colt, C. Wolter, N. Bekiroglu, D. Camann, P. Hartge, and J. R. Nuckols. 2006. Proximity to crops and residential exposure to agricultural herbicides in Iowa. *Environmental Health Perspectives* 114(6):893–897.

Young, A. L. 2007. *Public statement to the Committee on Making Best Use of the Agent Orange Exposure Reconstruction Model*, Meeting 2, April 30–May 1, Washington, DC.

Young, A. L., and M. Newton. 2004. Long overlooked historical information on Agent Orange and TCDD following massive applications of 2,4,5-T-containing herbicides, Eglin Air Force Base, Florida. *Environmental Science and Pollution Research* 11(4):209–221.

Young, A. L., J. A. Calcagni, C. E. Thalken, and J. W. Tremblay. 1978. *The toxicology, environmental fate, and human risk of Herbicide Orange and its associated dioxin*. OEHL TR-78-92, Final Report. Brooks Air Force Base, TX: U.S. Air Force Occupational and Environmental Health Laboratory.

Young, A. L., P. F. Cecil, and J. F. Guilmartin, Jr. 2004a. Assessing possible exposure of ground troops to Agent Orange during the Vietnam War: The use of contemporary military records. *Environmental Science and Pollution Research* 11(6):349–358.

Young, A. L., J. P. Giesy, P. D. Jones, and M. Newton. 2004b. Environmental fate and bioavailability of Agent Orange and its associated dioxin during the Vietnam War. *Environmental Science and Pollution Research* 11(6):359–370.

4

Data for Epidemiologic Studies of Vietnam Veterans

Chapter 3 examined the components of the Stellman team's herbicide exposure assessment model, including the geographic information system (GIS) and the Herbicide Exposure Assessment–Vietnam software tool. Chapter 3 also assessed the model's strengths and limitations in providing surrogates for exposure to herbicides sprayed in Vietnam. The model and its exposure metrics are welcome contributions to the effort to assess veterans' herbicide exposure, but other information must also be available to carry out epidemiologic studies.

This chapter addresses two categories of needed information: data on the likely location of individual study participants at particular times during their service in Vietnam, and health outcome information for these individuals. Important considerations and challenges are associated with gathering both types of information. Examining the availability, quality, and usefulness of existing information on Vietnam veterans permits consideration of some important factors that should be taken into account in planning for studies.

AVAILABLE TROOP LOCATION DATA

As described in previous chapters, the exposure assessment model makes use of a GIS consisting of two primary components: (1) a cleaned and documented georeferenced database abstracted from multiple types of military records providing information on herbicide spray missions during the Vietnam conflict, and (2) a database engine allowing information on locations of military units and their personnel to be entered and linked with the locations of spraying missions. To generate an exposure measure (a "hits" count, exposure opportunity index [EOI] score, or other exposure measure) for subjects in an epidemiologic study, it is necessary to have data on the location, in longitude and latitude, of study subjects for the duration of their deployment in Vietnam. However, because the locations of individuals were not recorded during their deployments, it is necessary to rely on the recorded locations of the units to which they were assigned.

Location Data Assembled by the Stellman Team

As a result of the work that has already been done, the committee found that at least some location-tracking information is available for more than 3,300 of the 4,778 U.S. Army units included in the Stellman team's databases. These databases also list 1,106 Air Force units, 22 Coast Guard units, 617 Marine Corps units, and 558 Navy units deployed to Vietnam. Location data have been tracked for all of the Air Force units, many Marine Corps units, and some Navy construction battalions and "brown water" units[1] (Stellman, 2007b). Location information for the remaining units and time periods is likely to be available but will have to be gathered through research of archival records (discussed below).

The Stellman team has made a distinction between stable units with missions that required only infrequent movement from base camp and mobile units that were frequently away from a base camp. In addition, some units were primarily stable but had elements that were mobile. Stellman and colleagues, with the assistance of the U.S. Army and Joint Services Records Research Center (JSRRC), developed location histories for 3,017 stable Army units, representing most of the combat arms support and combat support units assigned to Vietnam (Stellman and Stellman, 2003). According to the Stellman team (Stellman and Stellman, 2003), personnel serving in these units accounted for 80 percent of the troops in Vietnam.

Compiling location histories for mobile combat units is more challenging. Daily records for combat battalions may contain indications of multiple locations that reflect field positions of several companies and occasionally even platoons. The Stellman team has carried out preliminary cleaning and analysis of location data for more than 200 mobile Army combat units that were part of 55 battalions assigned to Military Region III of South Vietnam (also referred to as III Corps) between 1966 and 1969, a period and location of intense spraying (Stellman and Stellman, 2003). These location data had been gathered in the 1980s by the predecessor of

---

[1] "Brown water" Navy units operated in the rivers and deltas of Vietnam; "blue water" units operated in the open sea off the coast.

JSRRC on behalf of a study that had been planned (but was later cancelled) by the Centers for Disease Control and Prevention (CDC). The Stellman team plans to further clean and confirm location data for these units as part of a 3-year project that began in 2007 (see below; Stellman, 2007a). They also note that similar location data were collected for a set of Marine Corps units in conjunction with a Department of Veterans Affairs (VA) mortality study, and that with appropriate review those data could be added to the location databases (Stellman and Stellman, 2003).

The Stellman team (2003) carried out extensive quality control checks on their location data. For stable units, this included consultation with military experts and checks for erratic locations or movements that were considered too frequent. Major location changes detected in database entries were verified to avoid typographical or data-entry errors. The location data assembled for the mobile combat units were also evaluated in an effort to detect errors. When records showed multiple locations for a mobile unit on a single day (specified by Universal Transverse Mercator [UTM] values), the Stellman team calculated a weighted average (a "center-of-mass") and standard deviations for the UTM values. They paid special attention to cases in which the standard deviation was greater than 5 kilometers. In most cases corrections could be made, but some records were deleted from the database because evident errors could not be corrected. When their project ended in 2003, the Stellman team had not been able to complete their review of all suspect records or their review of data gaps, but they expressed confidence that many data problems could be resolved (Stellman and Stellman, 2003).

Concerns Regarding Troop Location Data

Although the locations of battalions may have little error, the aggregation of information at the battalion-level can lead to errors if those locations are attributed to individuals. Some uncertainty surrounds the assignment of a location to an individual on the basis of the reported location of the battalion-level unit (500 to 1,000 soldiers) or at best, a company-size unit (75 to 200 soldiers) to which he was assigned. Small units such as platoons were not always at the exact location of the larger units to which they were assigned, and the deviation of their location from that recorded for the larger unit (or the accuracy with which the unit's location was recorded) cannot now be determined. On the other hand, individuals' absences from their units are documented in records such as morning reports, which were generally prepared daily. Given the exigencies of combat, however, there are likely to be instances when a report was not created on a given day. Individuals' personnel files also may contain information about absences from the units to which they were assigned.

Some have raised other concerns about the location data for military units (e.g., Young et al., 2004; Ross and Ginevan, 2007). These critics claim that many relevant military records may be missing, incomplete, or reflect poor recordkeeping practices. They also point to military policies and Department of Defense (DoD) guidelines as evidence that the spray missions were planned with care to ensure that friendly forces were not in spray areas. However, a report by the General Accounting Office (GAO, 1979) estimated that for the period 1966–1969 about 5,900 marines were assigned to units that had been located within 0.5 kilometer of areas sprayed with Agent Orange on the same day. These troops were 2.7 percent of the 218,000 marines in Vietnam during 1966–1969. About 16,100 marines (7.4 percent) were within 0.5 kilometer of sprayed areas before the official DoD 4-week reentry period was over. The GAO (1979, p. 8) conclusion was that "DoD's contention that ground troops did not enter sprayed areas until 4 to 6 weeks afterward is inaccurate; the chances that ground troops were exposed to herbicide orange are higher than DoD previously acknowledged."

OBTAINING ADDITIONAL TROOP LOCATION DATA FROM MILITARY RECORDS

Even with the work already done and planned by the Stellman team, researchers using the exposure assessment model will inevitably need to abstract additional information from military records. The task is likely to include determining which individuals were assigned to units of interest, their dates of service and assignment histories, and, for units for which location information has not yet been gathered, following the units' movements over the period of interest. The Stellman team reported to the committee on their own experience with participants in a case-control study on amyotrophic lateral sclerosis (ALS) (Stellman, 2007c): Of the 384 units in which study participants served, complete tracking information had already been collected for 152 units and partial information for 102 units. For the remaining 130 units, they estimated that collection of unit location information would take roughly 30 days of work.

Access to Military Records

Military records from the Vietnam era include a mix of publicly accessible material and records still controlled by the individual military service branches. In either form, the records include handwritten notes and files, often stored on outdated media requiring specialized hardware to read. Most of the records are in paper form or on microfilm.

Three basic types of military records are likely to contain the kind of information that will be needed to develop location histories for military units or individual veterans:

1. The programmatic and operational records of military field organizations at various levels of the organizational hierarchy. These records (e.g., Army daily journals, Navy deck logs) contain reports on the locations and activities of troop units.

2. The personnel strength accounting records of military units, generally at the lowest level of the organizational hierarchy. These records include Army morning reports and rosters and Navy and Marine Corps muster rolls. Parallel records for Air Force units are only available through June 1966. Personnel strength accounting records identify the individuals assigned to the units that are the subjects of the programmatic and operational records.

3. The Official Military Personnel Files (OMPFs) of individual service members. These records contain demographic and other personal data on individuals and can provide dates of their unit assignments over the course of their military service.

The operational and programmatic records created by the U.S. Army in Vietnam have been accessioned by the National Archives and Records Administration (NARA). They are fully accessible to the public, with no administrative barriers or impediments to using them. For the most part, similar records created by the other branches of the armed services remain in the legal custody of those agencies and are generally available to researchers pursuant to a Freedom of Information Act (FOIA) request. Exceptions include deck logs of Navy ships and the Air Force Operation Ranch Hand records, both of which series have been accessioned by NARA. Some records, however, such as those created by intelligence organizations, may still retain security classifications and remain unavailable to those not having the appropriate security clearance.

Records in the second and third categories remain in the legal custody of the military services. Access to these records is restricted by provisions of the Privacy Act of 1974 (5 U.S.C. 552a) and the administrative rules promulgated under that act by each of the service departments. In general, the statute and rules limit access to the records to the individual subject of the record; his or her immediate next-of-kin (in the event of the subject's death); anyone specifically granted access by the subject of the record or, if the subject is deceased, by the next-of-kin; and the agency that created the record.

Access also is available to "routine users" of the record, which are entities designated by the creating agency and identified as having a legitimate need to access the record to conduct official business on behalf of the public.

Even with a routine user designation, it is necessary to request and receive permission for access to records for the specific purposes of any given study. Privacy rules also allow for access to the records by contractors of the creating agency, by other federal agencies and their contractors, and by private organizations "for purposes of conducting personnel and/or health-related research in the interest of the federal government and the public." These latter arrangements are ad hoc in nature, with access approval being granted on a case-by-case basis and inevitably involving a degree of uncertainty that is avoided when access is sought by an entity specifically designated a routine user of the records in the agency regulation.[2]

Access to personnel strength accounting records and OMPFs may be crucial for the completion of epidemiologic studies using the exposure assessment model. In the short term, based on the best information available from DoD and the military service departments, it would appear that investigators who seek access to personal data from records that document the service of Vietnam-era veterans would be best advised to

- contract directly with DoD or VA,
- contract with an organization that has been specifically designated by each of the service departments as a routine user of military personnel records, or
- enter into a collaboration with an investigator affiliated with any of these organizations.

However, the committee sees benefit in providing access to military records that remain in the legal custody of the services to support independent research, including work by investigators who are not under contract to DoD or VA, contingent on establishing and maintaining safeguards for privacy and for appropriate research use of the records. The committee urges VA to work with its sister agencies to make access to the relevant records feasible for independent researchers. If changes in the law are necessary to make this possible, the committee urges congressional attention to modifications in the law to improve appropriate access to records for research purposes.

---

[2]The committee notes that the National Academy of Sciences is cited by the Army, Navy, Marine Corps, and Air Force as an example of a "private organization" to which records containing personal data can be made available "for purposes of conducting personnel and/or health-related research in the interest of the Federal government and the public" (5 U.S.C. 552a; Department of the Air Force, 2000; Department of the Army, 2000; Department of the Navy, 2000; U.S. Marine Corps, 2000). The Navy regulation further names the National Research Council as a routine user of Navy privacy system records (5 U.S.C. 552a[b][3]; Department of the Navy, 2000).

Using Military Records to Gather Troop Location Information

Gaining legal access to military records is a necessary first step, but the challenges of gathering information from these records extend beyond that to the availability, quality, and usefulness of the information in the records. Table 4-1 lists the kinds of information that researchers may need, sources for those various types of information, and where the relevant military records are located. The committee notes that a compilation of information about the content, form, and location of combat and combat-related records from the Vietnam era, which was assembled in the mid-1970s (Carter et al., 1976), may also be useful to researchers attempting to work with any of these types of records.

Drawing upon committee expertise, input from experts provided at the committee's information-gathering sessions, and the experience of the Medical Follow-up Agency (MFUA) of the Institute of Medicine (IOM) in using military service records for epidemiologic studies, the committee identified several considerations to bear in mind in planning studies.

Personnel Strength Accounting Records

The Stellman team has done extensive work on identifying units that served in Vietnam, but epidemiologic studies will require information on the individuals who served in these units over time. This information can be gathered from the personnel strength accounting records of military units, which identify the individuals assigned to each unit.

Navy and Marine Corps muster rolls are stored at the National Archives facility in College Park, Maryland. Army morning reports and unit rosters are stored at NARA's National Personnel Records Center (NPRC) in St. Louis, Missouri. Also stored at NPRC are Air Force morning reports through June

TABLE 4-1 Types and Sources of Information for Developing Location Histories for Military Units or Personnel

Information Type	Source	Location
Individuals serving in a unit	Personnel strength accounting records of military units	NARA, College Park, Maryland NPRC, St. Louis, Missouri
Individual's history of unit assignments	Official Military Personnel Files	NPRC
Locations of units during deployment in Vietnam	Programmatic and operational records of military field organizations	NARA

NOTE: NARA, National Archives and Records Administration; NPRC, National Personnel Records Center.

1966. If the services grant permission to access the records at NPRC, records must be located and retrieved by NPRC staff, typically according to a schedule that is requested in advance through a formal contract. The records are on microfilm and must be reviewed in the NPRC Research Room. Alternatively, copies of the film maybe ordered from NPRC and shipped to researchers.

Official Military Personnel Files

When the identities of individual study subjects are known, researchers will need to access OMPFs to determine each individual's dates of entry into and exit from units during Vietnam service. Veterans' military personnel records are stored at NPRC in St. Louis, and as with the other records held there, they must be accessed through NPRC personnel and viewed on site.

Personnel files may sometimes be unavailable because they have been misfiled or are in use.[3] In carrying out data collection for their work, the Stellman team provided NPRC with a list of 6,393 names and Social Security numbers of veterans for whom they sought dates of service and unit assignment information. They received useful information on 91 percent of the individuals, but for 574 veterans the files were unavailable or the data abstracted by NPRC could not be used (Stellman and Stellman, 2003). A pilot study carried out as part of an IOM study of sailors exposed to test agents in the 1960s found that of a sample of 174 hard-copy personnel records requested, 32 of them (18 percent) were not available (IOM, 2007). Eight records were charged out for another use, and 24 could not be found.

The location of information on unit assignments within a service member's personnel file will vary with the branch of service. For Army files, the information in Vietnam-era records is summarized on a single card-stock form (DA Form 20) in the service member's file. A soldier whose military career extended over several periods of service may have more than one DA Form 20, but the forms are readily identifiable and are generally filed together in the record. Even so, a review of the entire file may be useful to ensure that a complete location history is compiled. Information on unit assignments for Marine Corps veterans may be available on a summary form. For those who served in the Navy, the information is likely to be clearly identified but distributed through the record. Some of the sources of information on assignment histories have been identified by the Stellman team (Stellman et al., 2003).

Careful plans should be made for the data abstraction process to ensure that information can be collected from the personnel records efficiently and in a usable form. Unit assignments can be designated in various ways, and

---

[3]A 1973 fire at the National Personnel Records Center had little impact on records of Vietnam-era veterans (see http://www.archives.gov/st-louis/military-personnel/fire-1973.html).

they will need to be recorded in a manner that will ensure that a consistent set of unit assignments can be generated. If researchers intend to make use of the unit location histories that the Stellman team has compiled, they will need to ensure that the information collected on individuals' unit assignments can be linked to the unit nomenclature used in the exposure assessment model. Researchers should also consider whether there is other information in the personnel records, such as demographic data or occupational duties, that they would want to have collected at the same time. The Stellman team's review of data abstraction work done by others suggested that errors were made with 9 to 10 percent of the records (Stellman and Stellman, 2003). As with any records-based research, it will be important to ensure that the personnel performing the data abstraction are well trained and that verification procedures are part of the data collection process.

Programmatic and Operational Records of Military Field Organizations

Although the Stellman team has assembled at least partial location histories for many military units, researchers may find it necessary to collect additional unit location information. As noted, information on Army units can typically be found in military records stored by NARA in College Park, Maryland, and information on other units has to be obtained through the individual service branches. Researchers seeking information at College Park must request specific unit records from the Archives staff, and only a limited number of archive boxes can be requested at one time. Retrieved records can be reviewed, scanned, or photographed onsite; records cannot be taken from the Archives building.

Abstracting information about locations of units over the time of their deployment is likely to be a challenging task to those unfamiliar with military recordkeeping. It can greatly benefit from a familiarity with military activities in Vietnam and typical means of recording those activities. Guidance in this task is available from such sources as a description of standard operating procedures prepared by a predecessor of the Army's JSRRC (Department of the Army, 1985) and a guide to the use of military records prepared by the Stellman team (Stellman et al., 2003).

The Army document describes daily journals as probably providing the most accurate record of unit activities, with a hierarchy of other information sources that can be consulted, including situation reports, intelligence summaries, lessons learned reports, after-action reports, and morning reports (Department of the Army, 1985). Many of these documents were produced at the battalion, brigade, and division levels. Similarly, the Stellman team's document describes the different types of primary information sources available and suggests appropriate strategies for finding unit locations. Figure 4-1 shows an excerpt from a daily journal.

\ DAILY STAFF JRNAL OR DUTY OFFICER'S LOG)	PAGE NO. 2	NO OF PGS				
ORGANIZATION OR INSTALLATION	LOCATION	PERIOD COVERED			
HHC, 3D BDE 1ST AIR CAV DIV	LZ EVANS, YD 540320	FROM		TO	
		HOUR 0001	DATE 4 Feb 68	HOUR 2400	DATE 4 Feb 68

ITEM NO	TIME IN	TIME OUT	INCIDENTS, MESSAGES, ORDERS, ETC	ACTION TAKEN	IN
24	1257		Fm Bde Scouts: fm 041130H - to 041200H: YD 644312 - 2 VC KIA, obs numerous spider holes along rd; YD 653- 313 ARVN outpost was over-run, many 60mm rds un-exploded; YD 608273 1 VC KIA many nu bunkers & trenches in area.		
25	1329		Fm 1-7: D Co at 1240H vic YD 553289, fd 1 60mm mortar rd. A Booby trap - pressure type detonater - they will dest it w/grenade.		
26	1258		Fm 1-7: A/26 YD 532335; C Co(-) YD 565305.	POSTED.	
27	1320		Fm 1-7: C (-) at 1300H vic YD 565302 fd a 105mm booby trap, will dest in place.		
28	1329		Fm 8 Engr: Minesweep tm which left Evans for PK 17, has been cplt. Tm heading N has not been cplt. Are held up by crater in road.		
29	1349		Fm 5-7: Med-evac for the 2 line 2 S fm C Co was cplt at 1340H.		
30	1350		Fm 1-7: In ref to D Co's previous rpt of finding a 60mm mortar rd booby trap: It was a 82mm mortar. It was dest in place & at same loc they fd a sign, made out of a piece of tin w/letters CAM. C Co rpts that the 105mm rd booby trap they fd had never been fired. It was a new rd. C Co at YD 563302 fd another booby trap which consisted of a can covered w/glass. Inside the can was a blasting cap & charge. It also had a trip wire leading fm it.		
31	1400		Fm 5-7: A Co YD 639273; C Co PK 17; D Co YD 636286; B Co LZ Jack.	INFO TO G3.	
32	1410		Fm 5-7: C Co at 1405H vic YD 650270, fd 1 psn believed to be an AW psn.		
33	1413		Fm 1-7: C Co YD 568302; D Co YD 547295; A/16 is at the drop zone; A/26 closed LZ Evans at 1358H.	POSTED.	
34	1415		Fm Maj Scudder 2-12: Ref 2 ammo re-supply alloys: 1st landed OKay - 2d rec hits & is leaking fuel. Is ret to this loc. Req a replacement for ship which was hit.		
35	1534		Fm 1-7: A/36 YD 515295; A(-) LZ Evans; B Co LZ Evans; C Co(-) YD 565310; D Co LZ Evans.	POSTED.	
36	1555		Fm 1-9: D/1-9 (Blues) YD 462399; D/1-9 (Red&White) YD 635295.	INFO TO G3.	
37	1603		Fm 1-7: A Co/46 is on mine sweep to the N (loc YD 460403).	POSTED.	
38	1610		Fm C/1-9: YD 527341, UH-1H rec 1 rd SA fire w/1 hit. (400' at 100 knots). Acft is flyable.		
39	1625		Fm 1-9: Between Hue - Phu Bai & the coast a UH-1B/C rec fire & took some hits in cockpit, (still flyable) no further details at this time.		
40	1630		Fm 5-7: 5-7 CP was lifted to PK 17 around 1600H.	INFO TO G3.	
41	1640		Fm 1-9: Ref acft firing at 1625H vic was 4 miles SE of Hue Phu Bai & altitude 600' - speed approx 100 knots.		

TYPED NAME AND GRADE OF OFFICER OR OFFICIAL ON DUTY / SIGNATURE

FIGURE 4-1 A Daily Journal excerpt. The excerpt illustrates a record of the activities of A, C, and D companies of the Headquarters and Headquarters Company, Third Brigade, First Air Cavalry Division, over a 4-hour period on February 4, 1968. Locations are specified using UTM coordinates, which are given as two letters followed by six numerals, for example YD 644312.
SOURCE: Department of the Army, 1968.

The size of the unit for which detailed location information is available varies, and the quality of units' recordkeeping is not consistent (Shaughnessy, 1991; Boylan, 2007). Larger units (e.g., battalions) are generally more likely to have records of their daily locations than are smaller units such as companies. The Stellman team (Stellman et al., 2003) notes that for Army infantry and cavalry units, which are likely to be highly mobile, detailed locations can be found only for battalions or squadrons (100 to 1,000 men). However, these records often can be used to determine the locations of units' component companies or troops and, in some cases, also can be used to determine the locations of their component platoons. Determining the locations of independent companies or troops is more difficult and time-consuming, and many times not possible.

Other Sources of Location and Personnel Information

The Stellman team (Stellman and Stellman, 2003) suggests that Vietnam veterans themselves be considered for sources of information such as maps and photographs that may aid in locating individuals or units. In addition, several military units and veterans organizations have compiled histories that may include troop locations, combatant names, and dates of service. Although these data vary in completeness, coverage, and accuracy, they may serve as a source of confirmatory and supplementary information.

Committee Comment on Collection of Troop Location Data

Despite some of the limitations of the available data resources for troop locations and the challenges in assembling additional data, the committee considers the approach the Stellman team took toward development of their unit location database to be reasonable, and it has some confidence that their approach would be successful. However, as the committee gained an understanding of the procedures necessary to gather location data for military units and the inherent challenges of those procedures, it had increasing concerns regarding the ability of typical academic researchers to carry out this work without the benefit of expertise in military records. The committee agrees with the guidance given by the Stellman team that "it is essential that those with specific experience and knowledge of military records and military terminology be involved in the research" (Stellman et al., 2003). In their work the Stellman team benefited from interaction and collaboration with what is now JSRRC. But the capacity of JSRRC to respond to requests may be limited (see GAO, 2006), without additional resources. The Stellman team also cautions that for the high volume of records likely to be needed for a major epidemiologic study, the current method of record retrieval available to researchers using the NARA facility may not be practical. The Stellman team urges consideration of an arrangement that can draw upon the experience and skills of the JSRRC in using military records (Stellman et al., 2003). The committee concurs.

SOURCES OF HEALTH OUTCOME INFORMATION

To carry out a study examining potential associations between exposure to herbicides and health problems in Vietnam veterans, researchers will need information on individuals' health outcomes as well as troop locations. This section discusses sources of health information for Vietnam veterans and related access issues. Many of the challenges involved in gathering health outcome information for veterans are not unique to this population and should be familiar to epidemiologists carrying out studies on members of the civilian population.

Mortality Data

Information regarding mortality for an epidemiologic study is available from several sources. Complete information on deaths since 1979, including cause of death, is available for the U.S. population through the National Death Index, or NDI. Maintained by the National Center for Health Statistics, NDI is a computerized file of the death information available through each of the states' vital statistics offices (NCHS, 2007). Lists of potential study subjects can be compared with NDI entries to determine which subjects are deceased, their dates of death, and the states in which they died. Users are charged $0.15 for each year searched for each study subject. For example, records for 10,000 study subjects searched against 10 years would cost $15,000 ($0.15 × 10,000 × 10), plus a small user's fee. For large studies covering many years, the costs can be significant. For slightly higher fees, NDI (through "NDI Plus") can also be the source of information on cause of death, as recorded on death certificates.

A potentially useful source of mortality information specifically for U.S. veterans is VA's Beneficiary Identification and Record Locator Subsystem (BIRLS). The automated system identifies veterans and their beneficiaries who have received compensation, pension, education, and other VA benefits (Kang, 2007a). A 1996 study of deceased male veterans born between 1936 and 1955 (a proxy for Vietnam-era service) found BIRLS death ascertainment to be roughly 90 percent complete (Page et al., 1996). A more recent study, however, suggested that BIRLS death reporting may be only 77 percent complete (Sohn et al., 2006) and concluded that BIRLS mortality ascertainment is, by itself, too incomplete for research use.

Information on veterans' deaths can also be obtained from the Social Security Administration's Death Master File (SSA DMF), which contains records for some 65 million deaths reported to the Social Security Administration (NTIS, 2007). The file can be purchased by researchers, along with quarterly updates. A recent study suggests that ascertainment of veterans' deaths is roughly 92 percent complete in the SSA DMF (Sohn et al., 2006).

Another source of mortality information for older veterans is the Medicare Vital Status file, which is maintained by the Centers for Medicare and Medicaid Services (CMS). The primary source of information for this file is the SSA DMF, but it is updated with information from other sources, including Medicare claims data (Sohn et al., 2006). Sohn et al. (2006) found the Medicare Vital Status file to be 83.2 percent complete in their sample of veterans, and for veterans enrolled in Medicare it was the most accurate and complete (99 percent) of all single sources of death information evaluated.

Studies assessing mortality are likely to benefit from using more than one of the information sources. Access to the NDI, SSA DMF, and Medicare Vital Status file is readily available to researchers, while access to VA's BIRLS database is more limited.

Morbidity Data

Obtaining information for studying morbidity of Vietnam veterans is more problematic than obtaining information about mortality. Because of the dispersed nature of health care in the United States, Vietnam veterans receive care from many types of providers and care systems. The committee focused its attention on the strengths and weaknesses of VA and Medicare data and data systems, which it saw as two promising sources of morbidity data for Vietnam veterans. Researchers could also explore other resources such as state cancer registries and hospital discharge datasets. In addition, if data are needed on the cumulative incidence of a condition, it may be necessary to obtain information on veterans' medical histories and medical care during military service.

VA Databases

Morbidity data are available from VA from three primary sources: the Patient Treatment File (PTF), which contains data on persons who received inpatient care at VA facilities; the Outpatient Clinic File (OPC), which similarly contains records for outpatient care given at VA facilities; and a set of health registries (see Box 4-1). VA researchers have used the PTF as the starting point for case-control studies of Vietnam veterans (e.g., Kang et al., 1986; Dalager et al., 1991; Mahan et al., 1997). The study populations assembled for these studies are discussed in Chapter 5 as potential popu-

BOX 4-1
VA Health Information Databases

BIRLS

The Beneficiary Identification and Record Locator Subsystem (BIRLS) is an automated system identifying veterans and their beneficiaries who have received compensation, pension, education, or other VA benefits (Kang, 2007a). The database has more than 44 million records and includes an initial record for each person discharged from military service since the early 1970s. The database contains information that includes veterans' names, social security numbers, dates of birth and death, gender, periods and branches of service, and current location of claim folders. One of the most frequent research uses of the BIRLS database is in identifying deceased veterans for mortality studies (Page et al., 1996; Boyko et al., 2000).

Patient Treatment File

The Patient Treatment File (PTF) contains information on inpatient records from each discharge from a VA hospital facility since 1970. Data are updated every 2 weeks. Currently, the database captures approximately 400,000 discharges annually, down from a peak of about 1 million annually in the late 1980s (Kang, 2007a). The PTF's demographic data is complete except for address, but information on military history is not considered reliable. For each discharge, up to 10 different diagnostic codes are recorded, including an indication of the diagnosis most responsible for the length of stay. The PTF can be used as a sampling frame to identify potential subjects for case-control studies. It can also be used to assess health care utilization or morbidity for selected cohorts of veterans. However, there is no quality control on the data, which are subject to the errors that are typical in medical records (Kang, 2007a).

Outpatient Clinic File

The Outpatient Clinic File (OPC) contains records from visits to outpatient VA clinics. Records prior to 1997 contain only basic utilization data. The newer records include information for each clinic stop during a patient visit and include demographic information and up to 10 diagnostic and 15 procedural codes. In 2004, 4.9 million unique veterans were seen at VA outpatient centers (Kang, 2007a).

Health Registries

VA maintains various health registries. The Agent Orange Registry includes records for nearly 409,000 veterans who have identified themselves as having concerns about medical problems related to exposure to Agent Orange and who have undergone physical examinations (Kang, 2007a). The Cancer Registry is compiled from cancer registries maintained at each VA facility. It contains records on all veterans receiving a diagnosis of cancer within the VA medical system. VA also has registries of veterans diagnosed within the VA system with other conditions, including ALS, multiple sclerosis, and hepatitis C.

lations for studies based on applications of the Stellman team's exposure assessment model.

It is estimated that 20 percent of veterans from the Vietnam War era receive at least a portion of their medical care through the VA system (VA, 2001). Among a sample of veterans between 55 and 64 years of age, for example, 7.6 percent reported receiving health care only from VA sources and 12.7 percent reported using both VA and non-VA health care sources (VA, 2001). Despite Vietnam-era veterans' limited use of VA health care services, VA records are likely to provide the largest proportion of health information on Vietnam veterans available from any single source.

Use of VA health care data for epidemiologic studies is problematic, as it is difficult to estimate the population at risk. For example, if there were no record of an individual having received medical treatment from VA, it could mean that person was healthy or was receiving medical care elsewhere. Users of VA data must consider that the Vietnam veterans who use VA medical care are probably not representative of the population of Vietnam veterans as a whole. An analysis of veterans overall found that those who did not use VA health care services had higher incomes, more education, and better health status than those who relied entirely or in part on VA health care (Nelson et al., 2007).

Access to VA's administrative databases, health care information, and medical records is generally restricted to researchers who are part of the VA system (employed at least 5/8 time by VA). Should access issues be overcome for other researchers, the VA resources described in Box 4-1 may be of interest to them, taking into account the constraints discussed above.

Medicare Claims Data

As more Vietnam veterans reach the age of 65 and become eligible for Medicare health insurance, Medicare data may prove increasingly useful as a source of information on health status for this population. A 2001 survey of veterans found that 96 percent of those who were age 65 or older were enrolled in Medicare (VA, 2001). Table 4-2 shows that something approaching 30 percent of the nearly 3 million veterans listed in VA's Vietnam Veteran Roster were eligible for Medicare in 2007. Within the next 10 years more than 90 percent of them will be eligible.

Under a data-sharing agreement with CMS, VA receives Medicare data for enrolled veterans each year (Sohn et al., 2006). Other researchers can obtain data from the Medicare system on the demographics of enrollees and on billing claims for beneficiaries' Medicare-eligible fee-for-service encounters. About 85 percent of Medicare coverage is accounted for by fee-for-service claims (as opposed to managed care) (CMS, 2007). The claims data contain information on diagnoses, treatments, costs, lengths of stay,

TABLE 4-2 Distribution of Veterans Included in the Vietnam Veteran Roster, by Year of Birth[a]

Birth Year	Number of Veterans	Percent	Cumulative Percent
1900–1910	1,029	< 0.1	< 0.1
1911–1915	2,584	0.1	0.1
1916–1920	15,985	0.6	0.7
1921–1925	36,415	1.3	2.0
1926–1930	97,253	3.5	5.4
1931–1935	186,874	6.6	12.1
1936–1940	200,061	7.1	19.2
1941–1945	475,397	16.9	36.1
1946–1950	1,539,984	54.7	90.8
1951–1955	252,917	8.9	99.7
1956–1957	7,532	0.3	100.0

[a]Based on the 2,816,031 veterans in the roster with a date of birth recorded.
SOURCE: Modified from Kang, 2007b.

and dates of service for every ambulatory visit and hospital stay covered by Medicare.

Demographic data can be obtained through the Vital Status File, as noted above, and a Denominator File, which includes all beneficiaries enrolled in a given year. Claims data are stored separately for different settings in which care is provided, including inpatient, outpatient, skilled nursing facility (SNF), and hospice care. A separate record exists for each service for which a payment claim was filed. Records on inpatient and SNF care are also available in a form that links all services for a given stay.

Access to individually identifiable CMS data is limited by Privacy Act provisions. Data can be made available to researchers upon approval of formal requests for specific study purposes (ResDAC, 2007b). To obtain data on specific individuals, researchers must submit Social Security numbers or other specified identifying information that will allow CMS to select records of interest. Although the claims files are complex and their primary purpose is not to support research studies, various academic groups have developed expertise in their use. In addition, the Research Data Assistance Center is funded by CMS specifically to aid government, academic, and nonprofit researchers in using Medicare (and Medicaid) data (ResDAC, 2007a).

CONCLUSIONS

From its review of the sources of data on troop locations and health outcomes that will be needed in order to apply the herbicide exposure assessment model in epidemiologic studies of Vietnam veterans, the committee reached the following conclusions:

1. It is generally possible to obtain useful data on individuals' unit assignments and unit locations. However, the processes of gaining permission for access to relevant military records and of collecting data for individuals is likely to be administratively difficult for many researchers, as well as time consuming and costly.

2. Assistance from experts in the location and interpretation of Vietnam-era military records is likely to be essential for effective collection of data from these sources.

3. With appropriate identifying information, mortality data for Vietnam veterans are readily and reliably available through the National Death Index and the Social Security Administration's Death Master File, while access to VA's Beneficiary Identification and Record Locator Subsystem is more limited. However, no single source of comprehensive morbidity data currently exists for these veterans. Within the next 10 years it should be possible to use Medicare records to obtain morbidity information for most Vietnam veterans.

4. Although VA has several databases that could contribute information about the health status of some Vietnam veterans, only about 20 percent of these veterans are receiving care from the VA, and access to VA data is typically restricted to VA researchers.

REFERENCES

Boyko, E. J., T. D. Koepsell, J. M. Gaziano, R. D. Horner, and J. R. Feussner. 2000. U.S. Department of Veterans Affairs medical care system as a resource to epidemiologists. *American Journal of Epidemiology* 151(3):307–315.

Boylan, R. 2007. *Accessing military unit records at the College Park Archives.* Oral presentation to the IOM Committee on Making Best Use of the Agent Orange Reconstruction Model, Meeting 2, April 30–May 1, Washington, DC.

Carter, G., J. W. Ellis, A. H. Peterson, J. H. Pierce, and J. S. Reiley. 1976. *User's guide to Southeast Asia combat data.* Document Number: R-1815-ARPA. Santa Monica, CA: RAND Corporation. http://rand.org/pubs/reports/2005/R1815.pdf (accessed November 1, 2007).

CMS (Centers for Medicare and Medicaid Services). 2007. 2007 Statistical supplement. *Health Care Financing Review.* http://www.cms.hhs.gov/MedicareMedicaidStatSupp/LT/list.asp (accessed October 19, 2007).

Dalager, N. A., H. K. Kang, V. L. Burt, and L. Weatherbee. 1991. Non-Hodgkin's lymphoma among Vietnam veterans. *Journal of Occupational Medicine* 33(7):774–779.

Department of the Air Force. 2000. Privacy Act of 1974; Notice to alter a system of records. *Federal Register* 65(199):60916–60918.

Department of the Army. 1968. *Daily staff journal or duty officer's log.* A, C, and D companies of the Headquarters and Headquarters Company, Third Brigade, First Air Cavalry Division. Photocopy.

Department of the Army. 1985. *ESG standard operating procedures: Steps in researching and tracking exposed combat units.* Washington, DC: U.S. Army and Joint Services Environmental Support Group.
Department of the Army. 2000. Privacy Act of 1974; Notice to alter a system of records. *Federal Register* 65(199):60918–60921.
Department of the Navy. 2000. Privacy Act of 1974; Notice to alter a system of records. *Federal Register* 65(199):60923–60925.
GAO (General Accounting Office). 1979. *U.S. ground troops in South Vietnam were in areas sprayed with Herbicide Orange.* FPCD-80-23. Washington, DC: U.S. Government Printing Office.
GAO (Government Accountability Office). 2006. *VA can improve its procedures for obtaining military records.* GAO-07-98. Washington, DC: U.S. Government Printing Office.
IOM (Institute of Medicine). 2007. *Long-term health effects of participation in Project SHAD (Shipboard Hazard and Defense).* Washington, DC: The National Academies Press.
Kang, H. K. 2007a. *Data resources within VA for an epidemiological study of Vietnam veterans.* PowerPoint presentation to the IOM Committee on Making Best Use of the Agent Orange Reconstruction Model, Meeting 2, April 30–May 1, Washington, DC.
Kang, H. K. 2007b. *Vietnam roster veterans: Demographic/military service characteristics.* Unpublished document submitted to the IOM Committee on Making the Best Use of the Agent Orange Reconstruction Model, July 11.
Kang, H. K., L. Weatherbee, P. Breslin, Y. Lee, and B. Shepard. 1986. Soft tissue sarcomas and military service in Vietnam: A case comparison group analysis of hospital patients. *Journal of Occupational and Environmental Medicine* 28(12):1215–1218.
Mahan, C. M., T. A. Bullman, and H. K. Kang. 1997. A case-control study of lung cancer among Vietnam veterans. *Journal of Occupational and Environmental Medicine* 39(8):740–747.
NCHS (National Center for Health Statistics). 2007. *National Death Index.* Division of Vital Statistics, Centers for Disease Control and Prevention. http://www.cdc.gov/nchs/r&d/ndi/what_is_ndi.htm (accessed September 18, 2007).
Nelson, K. M., G. A. Starkebaum, G. E. Reiber. 2007. Veterans using and uninsured veterans not using Veterans Affairs (VA) health care. *Public Health Reports* 122(1):93–100.
NTIS (National Technical Information Service). 2007. *Social Security Administration's Death Master File.* http://www.ntis.gov/products/pages/ssa-death-master.asp (accessed September 18, 2007).
Page, W. F., C. M. Mahan, and H. K. Kang. 1996. Vital status ascertainment through the files of the Department of Veterans Affairs and the Social Security Administration. *Annals of Epidemiology* 6(2):102–109.
ResDAC (Research Data Assistance Center). 2007a. *About us.* University of Minnesota. http://www.resdac.umn.edu/AboutUs/Index.asp (accessed October 8, 2007).
ResDAC. 2007b. *Medicare data available.* University of Minnesota. http://www.resdac.umn.edu/Medicare/data_available.asp (accessed October 8, 2007).
Ross, J. H., and M. E. Ginevan. 2007. *Points for the committee to consider when evaluating the Stellman model.* PowerPoint presentation to the IOM Committee on Making Best Use of the Agent Orange Reconstruction Model, Meeting 2, April 30–May 1, Washington, DC.
Shaughnessy, C. A. 1991. The Vietnam conflict: "America's best documented war"? *The History Teacher* 24(2):135–147.
Sohn, M. W., N. Arnold, C. Maynard, and D. M. Hynes. 2006. Accuracy and completeness of mortality data in the Department of Veterans Affairs. *Population Health Metrics* 4:2. http://www.pophealthmetrics.com/content/4/1/2 (accessed September 5, 2007).

Stellman, J. M. 2007a. *A data resource for the health and environmental consequences of the Vietnam War.* Unpublished document submitted to the IOM Committee on Making the Best Use of the Agent Orange Reconstruction Model, July 31.

Stellman, J. M. 2007b. *Responses to IOM 091407.* Unpublished document submitted to the IOM Committee on Making the Best Use of the Agent Orange Reconstruction Model, September 14.

Stellman, J. M. 2007c. *Separate modeling and reconstruction issues.* PowerPoint presentation to the IOM Committee on Making Best Use of the Agent Orange Reconstruction Model, Meeting 3, June 13–14, Washington, DC.

Stellman, J. M., and S. D. Stellman. 2003. *Contractor's final report: Characterizing exposure of veterans to Agent Orange and other herbicides in Vietnam.* Submitted to the National Academy of Sciences, Institute of Medicine, in fulfillment of Subcontract VA-5124-98-0019, June 30, 2003.

Stellman, J. M., R. Christian, S. D. Stellman, and F. Benjamin. 2003. Characterizing exposure to Agent Orange and other herbicides used in Vietnam: An epidemiologist's guide to useful military records (version 1.1 June 26, 2003). In *Contractor's final report: Characterizing exposure of veterans to Agent Orange and other herbicides in Vietnam.* By J. M. Stellman and S. D. Stellman. Submitted to the National Academy of Sciences, Institute of Medicine, in fulfillment of Subcontract VA-5124-98-0019, June 30, 2003.

U.S. Marine Corps. 2000. Privacy Act of 1974; Notice to alter a system of records. *Federal Register* 65(199):60914–60916.

VA (U.S. Department of Veterans Affairs). 2001. *National Survey of Veterans, 2001.* http://www1.va.gov/vetdata/docs/survey_final.htm (accessed August 28, 2007).

Young, A. L., P. F. Cecil, Sr., and J. F. Guilmartin, Jr. 2004. Assessing possible exposures of ground troops to Agent Orange during the Vietnam War: The use of contemporary military records. *Environmental Science and Pollution Research* 11(6):349–358.

5

Recommendations Regarding Epidemiologic Studies Using the Exposure Assessment Model

With this chapter the committee addresses the central question put to it by the Department of Veterans Affairs (VA): What are the best ways to use the Stellman team's herbicide exposure assessment model? The committee has concluded that epidemiologic studies applying the exposure assessment model should be considered, and in this chapter it discusses the potential contributions of and pitfalls in conducting such studies. The chapter discusses design and statistical considerations for studies, including the selection of health outcomes, potential study populations, and other criteria for optimal use of the model.

SHOULD STUDIES BE DONE USING THE STELLMAN TEAM'S MODEL?

The committee carefully considered the question of whether, given the shortcomings of the model in its current form and its inherent limitations even with further refinements, it holds promise for generating informative epidemiologic studies of herbicides and health among Vietnam veterans. The committee concluded that the answer is yes. It reached this decision based on two key considerations: (1) The exposure assessment model is applicable to the population of ultimate interest, namely Vietnam veterans; and (2) most previous studies of this population have been so severely limited with respect to exposure assessment that a more accurate yet imperfect method would advance the current understanding of whether herbicide exposure is associated with adverse health outcomes among Vietnam veterans. We recognize the logistical challenges to be faced in obtaining the needed model inputs (troop locations, unit membership), but based on ongoing and completed activities, these challenges appear to be surmountable. At the same time, while we appreciate the potential contributions from applying the model, we also believe that the best use of the model requires that its limitations be understood and considered when making decisions about the conduct of epidemiologic studies and particularly in interpreting the results of those studies.

CONTRIBUTIONS AND PITFALLS OF STUDIES USING THE MODEL

Studying the Population of Interest

Efforts to determine whether herbicide exposure among Vietnam veterans is associated with adverse health outcomes follow one of two approaches: (1) information from other populations, such as pesticide applicators or chemical production workers, is extrapolated to the experience of Vietnam veterans, an approach that has the advantage of being grounded in information about higher exposures that are more accurately characterized; or (2) studies are conducted among the Vietnam veterans themselves. The quality of the data and the statistical power of the first group of studies have been superior and will likely continue to generate more accurate information on herbicide exposure and health in general, particularly for dioxin, but the disadvantage of this approach is that there is an inevitable loss of information value when results are extrapolated from one population to another.

Furthermore, there is an inherent value in examining the issue of health effects of herbicide exposure in the Vietnam veterans themselves. The question posed by the VA is not the global one, "Is herbicide exposure associated with adverse health outcomes?", but rather the narrow one, "Did herbicide exposure affect the health of Vietnam veterans?" Because the herbicide exposures experienced by most Vietnam veterans are imperfectly characterized and presumably low compared with occupationally exposed populations, studies on these veterans can make only limited contributions to answering global questions regarding herbicides and health. However, studies on veterans have much greater potential than other studies to answer the narrower question about *their* exposure and *their* health. No other group has the confluence of exposures and exposure circumstances experienced by the Vietnam veterans, so given an adequate tool, it is important to ask the question in this group.

Improvement in Estimation of Exposure to Herbicides

Even with the advantage of studying exposure and health in the population of interest—Vietnam veterans—the Stellman team's herbicide exposure assessment model must offer incremental improvement over the methods of exposure assessment used in previous epidemiologic studies of Vietnam veterans if it is to be valuable. The committee concluded that it does offer such improvement. As noted in Chapter 3, many of the studies carried out in Vietnam veterans have relied on "service in Vietnam" as the exposure of interest in examining health outcomes. That approach in effect classifies all those who served in Vietnam as having been exposed to herbicides. Such studies have been able to make only limited contributions to the question of the health effects of exposure to herbicides in Vietnam because many of those considered "exposed" are likely to have had little or no contact with herbicides.

Accurate exposure classification is frequently the limiting factor in epidemiologic studies, particularly regarding environmental exposures. In simple terms, errors are introduced when those who are truly exposed are misidentified as unexposed (false negatives) and when those who are truly unexposed are misidentified as exposed (false positives). The shortcomings of an exposure assignment are sometimes explicit, as when service in Vietnam is used to define "exposure to herbicides" despite the certainty that many false positives will occur (unexposed veterans classified as exposed). In general, such errors, if independent of health outcomes, will tend to dilute any true associations between exposure and health. This will both bias measures of relative risk to be closer to the null value of 1.0 (i.e., no association) and increase the relative variance of estimated effects.

Although the actual proportion of Vietnam veterans who had potential for meaningful herbicide exposure is not known, given the temporal and geographic distribution of spraying, it seems likely that exposure was not universal or equal for all those who served. For instance, the Ranch Hand and Army Chemical Corps veterans, who handled the herbicides and presumably had higher exposures on average than other troops, can be studied with confidence as being exposed populations. But the challenge of addressing the broader population of Vietnam veterans remains. The Stellman team's model offers the possibility of establishing a gradient of exposure opportunity among the larger population of veterans.

In many instances requiring historical estimation of exposure, it is not possible to generate accurate, quantitative indices, and epidemiologists instead pursue a more modest goal of rank-ordering levels or probabilities of exposure. That is, without being able to specify a quantity of exposure, it is possible to place individuals into groups that have higher and lower levels or probabilities of exposure and examine patterns of health across those groups to determine whether the more highly exposed have excess risk of adverse health events. Such studies can identify associations even if they are unable to provide information on quantitative dose-response relationships.

The exposure assessment hierarchy discussed in Chapter 3 helps to illustrate both the potential contributions and the limitations of the model's exposure metrics. It is very likely that exposure metrics based on proximity to herbicide spraying provide a better estimate of exposure than does simple presence in Vietnam during certain years. The metrics are also likely to be an improvement over self-reported exposure to herbicides because individuals are unlikely to know when or if an area was sprayed before they arrived and could have mistaken insecticide spraying for herbicide spraying. Approximating target tissue doses in quantitative terms would be an ideal exposure measure, but it is unattainable. Thus, relative to an ideal, the Stellman team's herbicide assessment model is inherently limited, and even with major refinements will not approximate exposure classification based on precise individual doses. Still, there is incremental benefit in moving from poor to somewhat better approaches.

As a simple illustration of this point, consider the hypothetical results of a study that considers all veterans as exposed versus a study that correctly identifies some fraction of them as not exposed. For purposes of the example, assume that both exposure and disease are classified simply as either occurring or not occurring, and assume a true relative risk of 1.4. Our estimates of relative risk are accurate only if the classification of exposure is 100 percent accurate—that is, if all those who were presumed to be exposed truly were exposed, and all those presumed not to be exposed truly were not. With these assumptions, the value of correctly identifying at least some veterans as not exposed becomes clear: If all of those who served in Vietnam are classified as exposed (as many studies have done) when in truth only 20 percent of the troops who served were exposed, the relative risk would be calculated to be only 1.08—far less than the actual value. If exposure classification could be improved such that 80 percent of those designated as exposed actually were exposed (e.g., by applying an exposure classification model that more effectively isolates the troops who had potential herbicide exposure) and no one who was exposed was classified as not exposed (a false negative), the relative risk would be calculated as 1.32, which is much closer to the true value in this highly simplified example.

Although these results are hypothetical, they illustrate the principle that when the true risk among those exposed is only modestly increased, misclassification may well hinder identification of elevated risks. Improvements in estimation, even with error still present, would move the observed results in the direction of the value that would be obtained with no misclassification and be more likely to identify any associations between herbicide exposure and health that are truly present. By converting a dichotomous classification of exposure (yes/no) into an exposure opportunity score, even with measurement error, there are further gains in accuracy and statistical power. We expect that the exposure opportunity score, even if imprecise, will better identify the highly exposed individuals, improving the specificity[1] of the exposure assignment and therefore reducing the exposure misclassification bias. As noted above, improvements in specificity have the largest effect on reducing misclassification and attenuation of the relative risk (Flegal et al., 1986).

Although application of the Stellman team's model to estimate exposure can be expected to reduce some aspects of exposure misclassification, others will inevitably remain. It is possible that the Stellman team's exposure metrics and software tool could be improved with the incorporation of more detailed chemical fate and transport models. But moving from simple proximity to consideration of fate and transport will involve incorporating either more detailed assumptions or additional data regarding spray patterns, drift, meteorology, and ground cover, among others. Furthermore, the current model does not account for individual-level factors such as contact with contaminated plants and soil or consumption of tainted food or water, which may be an additional source of error in the exposure estimate. However, unlike the factors related to the flight path, which affect a whole unit's potential exposure, these individual-level factors influence how individual-level exposure is distributed around a group (unit) average. Therefore, omitting them should cause little or no bias, but it will generally tend to increase the confidence limits around the exposure estimates. In the absence of individual-level data on behavior or suspected systematic variations in individual behavior between locations or units, any additional modeling of exposure beyond fate and transport, such as different routes of exposure, is unlikely to appreciably change the rank order of exposure estimates.

The ultimate benefits of the Stellman team's exposure metrics depend, of course, on the reliability of the infrastructure around which they are built—the data on the location histories of spraying and military units or personnel. The committee concluded that the infrastructure is sufficiently reliable to justify use of the data, as long as sources of potential exposure misclassification are recognized. In particular, the documentation of herbicide spraying by fixed-wing aircraft appears to be more complete than that for the spraying by helicopters and ground equipment. In addition, analyses have shown high soil contamination with 2,3,7,8-tetrachlorodibenzo-p-dioxin (TCDD) at some former military bases (Dwernychuck

---

[1] In this context, specificity refers to how well truly unexposed people are classified as unexposed.

et al., 2002; Dwernychuck, 2005; Hatfield Consultants and Office of the National Steering Committee 33, MNRE, 2007), suggesting spills or other discharges of herbicide that would not be reflected in the spraying data. As a result, service members may have herbicide exposures that cannot be captured by the model's exposure metrics. Another consideration is that many of the herbicides used in Vietnam, or products similar to them, were also in widespread use at lower concentrations in the United States beginning before the Vietnam War, so veterans may have had some exposure to them and any TCDD contaminants before or after their military service. TCDD and other dioxins have also been present in the United States since the Vietnam War as chemical contaminants or byproducts of combustion and manufacturing processes.

The exposure sources that are not captured by the model would result in underestimation of herbicide exposures and the potential for false negatives—people designated as not exposed by the model who were in fact exposed to herbicides. If this exposure were randomly distributed across the study population, it would be expected to bias the relative risk toward the null, making true associations of health effects with herbicide sprayed from fixed-wing aircraft more difficult to discern.

Interpretation of Studies Using the Model

The committee was also concerned with how the results of studies of Vietnam veterans using the Stellman team's model should be interpreted, given the strengths and limitations of the approach. For established associations between herbicide exposure and health outcomes, finding a positive association in a study that applies this model to Vietnam veterans would provide evidence in support of the veterans having experienced health problems as a result of herbicide exposure. It would also add credibility to the ability of the model to classify exposure. On the other hand, interpreting a study that failed to find such associations would be much more challenging. In fact, at least four interpretations would be possible: (1) an association is truly present in the population, but the model failed to capture herbicide exposure with sufficient accuracy for the association to be detected; (2) study subjects were accurately assigned to exposure categories, but their herbicide exposure was at levels that are not associated with the health outcome; (3) study subjects' exposures are associated with such small levels of risk that they are not detectable using epidemiologic methods; or (4) the presumption that herbicides truly cause the health outcome studied is in error.

Note that these explanations pertain to the use of the model specifically to evaluate herbicide exposure and the health of Vietnam veterans. A separate issue is the contribution such studies might make to broader questions concerning the effects of herbicides on health. In those cases where there is a sizable body of high-quality epidemiologic research based on large populations with relatively high exposures, the incremental benefit of studies of herbicides and health among veterans would be small, given their relatively low and imperfectly documented herbicide exposure. Even with improvements in exposure assignment, their experience is less readily documented than that of some other groups that have already been studied.

On the other hand, where the current body of research on specific herbicides and health outcomes is less extensive—which is often the case for health outcomes other than cancer—the application of the Stellman team's exposure assessment model to Vietnam veterans does hold potential for advancing the larger body of knowledge concerning herbicides and health. That is, where the baseline level of information is lower, studies on Vietnam veterans may advance knowledge despite the known limitations in exposure levels and measurement. The ongoing research by the Stellman team addressing herbicides and amyotrophic lateral sclerosis (ALS) is one example of such a situation, as there has been a limited amount of work done on this topic to date. But any new associations observed in studies carried out using the model in Vietnam veteran populations will need to be confirmed in other herbicide-exposed populations.

Applying the model to approximate TCDD exposure is especially problematic. The variable (and unknown) concentrations of TCDD across herbicide batches make even a perfectly accurate assignment of proximity to spraying of limited value as a TCDD exposure proxy. The CDC (1988, 1989) Agent Orange study, which included only 646 Vietnam veterans, all of whom served no more than 1 year in Vietnam, is the most comprehensive study of veterans' serum TCDD levels performed to date. It found that serum TCDD levels in veterans who served in Vietnam were similar to those of veterans who did not serve there, but the study may not have captured a sufficient number of the most highly exposed soldiers. It is unlikely that meaningful new studies of TCDD levels in serum can be performed in the future because of the long period since the end of the war. This evidence and other studies (e.g., CDC, 1988; Mocarelli et al., 1991; Pirkle and Houk, 1992; Michalek et al., 1996; Sweeney et al., 1997–1998) suggest that the TCDD exposure of many Vietnam veterans was lower than that of other groups that have been studied epidemiologically, such as Air Force Ranch Hand personnel, herbicide production workers, or some of the residents of Seveso, Italy (e.g., those in Zone A). For this reason, studies of Vietnam veterans are not likely to contribute much to the overall knowledge of TCDD and health, regardless of how accurate the methods of exposure classification might become.

In summary, epidemiologic studies that use the Stellman team's exposure model have the potential to be informative about the health of Vietnam veterans, but they should not necessarily be expected to offer additional insight into the effects of TCDD at the toxicologic level because of inherent limitations in the accuracy of individual exposure assignment. However, the committee does see a possibility that more might be learned about the long-term health effects of exposure to the other herbicides that have not been as extensively studied and that were more consistent in composition.

GENERAL CONSIDERATIONS FOR CONDUCTING STUDIES

To make the best use of the Stellman team's exposure assessment model and produce meaningful epidemiologic findings for Vietnam veterans, several issues need to be considered that bear on the feasibility of studies and the information value of their results.

Representativeness of Vietnam Veterans

The committee has assumed that the main purpose of conducting studies using the exposure assessment model is to learn more about if and how Vietnam veterans' health was affected by herbicide spraying. Given that assumption, then study populations should reflect in a general way the breadth of experience of Vietnam veterans. And because the goal is to produce findings that would be applicable to all those who served, research should encompass the spectrum of experiences of potentially exposed troops. While formal random sampling is not necessary, broad representation is needed. Furthermore, oversampling of those most likely to have been exposed to herbicides would be helpful in enhancing statistical power. Specific candidate populations for study are considered below.

Broad Range of Health Outcomes

Research addressing proximity to spraying and health outcomes should provide a comprehensive view of the health of veterans and thus address a wide range of health outcomes. Studying outcomes believed to be related to herbicide exposure is of interest, because finding such associations in the veteran population would support the supposition that their exposures were high enough to produce health effects and that the exposures were represented by the model with sufficient accuracy for those effects to be detected. Addressing a wide range of health outcomes also has advantages in terms of efficiency. Depending on the sources of health outcome information, when information on one health outcome is gathered, it may not take much additional work to gather information on other outcomes.

In the most recent review by the Institute of Medicine (IOM) Committee on Veterans and Agent Orange (IOM, 2007), sufficient evidence for an association[2] with exposure to herbicides has been reported for the following conditions: chloracne, chronic lymphocytic leukemia, Hodgkin's disease, non-Hodgkin's lymphoma, and soft tissue sarcoma. Limited or suggestive evidence of an association was reported for laryngeal cancer; cancer of the lung, bronchus, or trachea; prostate cancer; multiple myeloma; AL amyloidosis; early-onset transient peripheral neuropathy; porphyria cutanea tarda; hypertension; Type 2 diabetes mellitus; and, in the offspring of exposed people, spina bifida.

Studies would also be of value for health outcomes that have even weaker evidence for an association with herbicide exposure. Among these are the health outcomes currently classified by IOM committees reviewing the literature on herbicides and health as having "inadequate or insufficient evidence" to determine an association with herbicide exposure. The most recent IOM review (IOM, 2007) includes in this category numerous types of cancer as well as lupus, stroke, and movement disorders, such as Parkinson's disease. Breast cancer is also in this category, but studying it poses special challenges because of the small number of women who served in Vietnam.[3]

In selecting health outcomes for study, researchers may want to take into account the ability of the Stellman team's exposure assessment software to generate separate exposure metrics for each of the herbicides used in Vietnam, including the arsenical cacodylic acid of Agent Blue and picloram in Agent White. The biennial reviews carried out by IOM contain careful reviews of the toxicologic and epidemiologic literature on the herbicides and can offer a source of guidance on outcomes of potential interest. As noted above, the contributions that the model can make to advancing general knowledge of herbicides and health depend to a great extent on the baseline level of understanding. Therefore, research on less extensively studied herbicides and health outcomes holds more promise for advancing

---

[2]Conclusions from the IOM reviews of evidence concerning associations between herbicides and health outcomes fall primarily into one of three categories (IOM, 2007): (1) *Sufficient evidence of an association* means that a positive association has been observed in studies in which chance, bias, and confounding can be ruled out with reasonable confidence. (2) *Limited or suggestive evidence of an association* means that the body of evidence suggests an association, but chance, bias, or confounding cannot be confidently ruled out. (3) *Inadequate or insufficient evidence to determine an association* means that available studies have inconsistent findings or are of insufficient quality or statistical power to support a conclusion regarding the presence of an association.

[3]The IOM committee that conducted the most recent review of the evidence concerning herbicides and health outcomes was unable to reach consensus on the classification for breast cancer, melanoma, and ischemic heart disease (IOM, 2007). As a default, these three conditions were assigned to the category of "inadequate or insufficient evidence" of an association rather than to the category of "limited or suggestive evidence," which indicates somewhat stronger support for an association.

general knowledge of the health effects of a herbicide than does additional research on topics already well studied.

It may also be worthwhile to consider whether proximity to herbicide spraying can serve as a proxy for combat stress or other factors that might be relevant in studying such outcomes as suicide, posttraumatic stress disorder, and cardiovascular disease.

Completeness and Timeliness of Health Data

Studying the relationship between herbicide exposure in Vietnam and health outcomes that are often not fatal, such as diabetes or prostate cancer, might be strengthened by using data on morbidity in addition to mortality data. In these cases it is important to determine health outcomes accurately and comprehensively both for the sake of precision (to maximize the number of cases) and for validity (to ensure that the measures of association between herbicide exposure and health are accurate). The issue of statistical power is addressed more fully below, but to the extent that there is under-ascertainment of health outcomes in veterans, it seems likely that the degree of under-ascertainment will be unrelated to exposure opportunity scores, meaning that there will be either no bias or a bias towards the null in relative measures of association.

As discussed in Chapter 4, researchers will face challenges in accessing morbidity data stemming from the dispersed nature of health care in the United States. These challenges are not unique to studies of veterans, however, and both the VA and Medicare systems are leading possibilities for consideration.

With Vietnam veterans reaching older ages and their overall likelihood of health problems therefore increasing, studies should aim to ascertain health status up to recent time periods. Reanalysis of health outcome data that were collected for past studies has the appeal of being somewhat simpler than initiating a new study: The principal task becomes developing location histories for the study subjects whose health outcome data have already been collected. But, depending on how long ago the study was originally conducted, this approach would miss the opportunity to incorporate additional, more recent data on the study population's health experience.

Statistical Power

Proposed studies will need to have adequate statistical power to detect an association between health effects and exposure to herbicides in Vietnam, if in fact one exists. Statistical power depends on several factors: the risk of error considered acceptable in concluding that no effect is present, the risk of concluding that an effect is present when it is not, the size of the effect detected relative to the amount of variability in the population, and the size of the sample. The smaller the effect anticipated, the larger the sample size needed to reliably detect it.

The committee expects that a very large study population (in the tens of thousands) will be needed to conduct cohort studies of health effects in relation to Vietnam veterans' exposure to herbicide spraying, particularly for relatively rare outcomes such as soft tissue sarcoma or ALS. For cancer endpoints, where we have the most prior knowledge, three factors suggest that the magnitude of the effect (e.g., the relative risk) is likely to be small in studies of Vietnam veterans: (1) the excess of cancer was relatively small in many previous studies of more highly exposed populations, including those involved in Operation Ranch Hand and even pesticide production workers and applicators (see IOM, 2007); (2) the exposure to herbicides among the majority of Vietnam veterans is likely to be low relative to these previously studied occupational and environmental cohorts; and (3) the degree of accuracy of the model in representing differences in veterans' exposure is uncertain. For these reasons, studies should be designed to have sufficient power to detect even modest effects.

Confounding

Another major consideration in designing an epidemiologic study to evaluate possible adverse health effects of herbicide exposures in Vietnam veterans is the need to control for potential confounders, such as tobacco, alcohol, or drug consumption. Some Vietnam veterans, particularly among those with posttraumatic stress disorder, are likely to have had high rates of alcohol or drug use (e.g., McFall et al., 1992). It is also possible that exposure to combat stress might be correlated with exposure to spraying operations.

Confounding may be controlled by including potential confounding factors in the statistical analyses, for example, or by restricting analyses to veterans with similar potential for exposure to combat-related stress and with similar socioeconomic backgrounds (Stellman and Stellman, 2003).

Analytic Approaches

Researchers planning to use the Stellman team's exposure metrics in an epidemiologic study should recognize and seek ways to mitigate the impact of the many unmeasured determinants of exposure operating at the unit level and affecting individuals within units. The model's predictions for unit exposures are subject to error, and statistical methods to account for such limitations at the level of unit assignment and individuals within units merit further consideration and refinement. Multilevel (or hierarchical) models would constitute one approach to incorporating measurement error into the analysis (e.g., see Dominici et al., 2000; Greenland, 2000). A different approach using Monte Carlo maximum likelihood methods has recently been successfully applied to estimate the impact of errors in exposures on an analysis of studies of radiation workers (Stayner et al., 2007).

Need for Sensitivity Analysis

Studies of veterans based on the Stellman team's exposure model should include analyses to assess how sensitive the estimated association between the measured exposure opportunity and specific health outcomes is to various sources of uncertainty as well as to the various assumptions made in specifying the precise form of the model. In Chapter 3 the committee discussed the need for sensitivity analyses to summarize the variability in the model's exposure metrics under different assumptions underlying the exposure opportunity model. The results of the sensitivity analyses for measurement of exposure opportunity would provide input into sensitivity analyses carried out during epidemiologic studies. These results will provide ranges and distributions of exposure opportunities that may be included in statistical estimates such as rate ratios and logistic regression parameters. By systematically varying the exposure opportunity metric, researchers can obtain a range or distribution of the estimated risks associated with the exposure, which reflects the implications of the underlying uncertainty in the assumptions of the Stellman team's model.

Although a "gold standard" measure of exposure is highly desirable for estimating the bias in a relative risk estimate due to exposure measurement error, it is not necessary for obtaining a plausible range of relative risk estimates associated with different exposure measures obtained from the model's sensitivity analysis. The examination of this range of relative risk estimates will increase the likelihood of identifying associations of potential importance, and it will also help to reflect more accurately the uncertainty inherent in all of the indices of herbicide exposure.

Providing Access for Independent Investigators

By taking full—and appropriate—advantage of their unique access to and knowledge of data sources on veterans' health, VA's intramural investigators have been prominent in investigations of relationships between veterans' exposures during the Vietnam War and the health effects they have experienced. However, the committee sees important benefits in opening research opportunities to the broader scientific community through contracts or collaborations. Adopting this broader approach to research on veterans' health should enhance the potential for identifying novel, creative applications of the Stellman team's model. In addition, public acceptance of and trust in the findings may be enhanced if the research processes are made more accessible.

The committee recognizes that, as described in Chapter 4, accessing the needed service records and health outcomes data presents substantial logistical challenges for most investigators outside VA. Because the committee sees value in trying to improve the ability of a broad range of researchers to work with those data resources, it recommends that VA work with the Department of Defense (DoD), the individual branches of the armed forces as necessary, and the National Archives and Records Administration (NARA) in at least two specific areas: first, to facilitate health research uses of military records that are subject to access barriers arising from privacy laws; and, second, to help arrange for DoD and NARA staff with appropriate expertise to aid researchers in the location and interpretation of military records for health research uses.

Promoting Refinements and Extensions of Epidemiologic Studies Using the Stellman Team's Model

The committee was very encouraged to learn that Dr. Jeanne Stellman has received funding from the National Library of Medicine (NLM) for a 3-year project to support work on—and to facilitate researchers' access to—the exposure assessment model and the data on herbicide spraying and unit and troop locations that have been assembled to date (Stellman, 2007a). Assembling these data has required a substantial effort, and making them available to others via a planned website can be expected to remove a major obstacle to their broader use. The committee wants to encourage those who conduct studies applying the Stellman model not only to address meaningful epidemiologic questions but also to follow the example set by the Stellman team in contributing building blocks for reanalyses and refinements by others.[4]

This approach is clearly in the spirit of reproducible epidemiologic research proposed by Peng and colleagues (2006). Their criteria for reproducibility call for "datasets and software to be made available to the scientific community for (1) verifying published findings; (2) conducting alternative analyses of the same data; (3) eliminating uninformed criticisms that do not stand up to existing data; and (4) expediting the interchange of ideas among investigators" (Peng et al., 2006, p. 783).

A study is considered reproducible when it satisfies the criteria in Table 5-1.

---

[4]The Stellman team considers all of the software code that they have developed to be open source and will provide it to researchers upon request (Stellman, 2007b).

TABLE 5-1 Criteria for Reproducible Epidemiologic Research

Research Component	Requirement
Data	Analytical data set is available.
Methods	Computer code underlying figures, tables, and other principal results is available in a human-readable form. In addition, the software necessary to execute the code is available.
Documentation	Adequate documentation of the computer code, software environment, and analytical data set is available to enable others to repeat the analyses and conduct other similar ones.
Distribution	Standard methods of distribution are employed for others to access the software, data, and documentation.

SOURCE: Peng et al., 2006. Reproduced with permission.

Peng et al. (2006) make a distinction between "measured" data and "analytical" data. The measured data are raw data, such as digital images of the military records extracted from the archives. These measured data are processed to create analytical data, such as the geocoded HERBS file and other individual electronic databases. The analytical data in turn serve as the input to analysis programs to produce such outputs as the exposure metrics of hits or the exposure opportunity index (EOI). Making available the data in the cleaned and checked HERBS file along with the source code and documentation for arriving at the calculated an exposure measures (hits and EOI) for each grid location, as the Stellman team plans to do, would go far toward making the workings of the herbicide exposure assessment model reproducible by other researchers. Similarly, their plans to make publicly available the compiled, cleaned, and checked databases of unit locations already developed would facilitate the work of future researchers.

The committee sees such steps as important for those who use the exposure assessment model in epidemiologic studies, and it urges researchers, including those at VA, to promote the reproducibility of studies conducted using the Stellman team's model. The work that they carry out to determine unit locations and calculations used to arrive at exposure indices should be documented and made available, ideally through the Internet and potentially via the resources being developed under Dr. Stellman's NLM grant, to enable others to repeat the analyses. Any extension or refinement of the model should also be documented so that others can evaluate and build on the work.

TYPES OF STUDIES FOR CONSIDERATION

Specific study designs must be determined on the basis of the questions chosen for investigation, but, in principle, either cohort or case-control studies may be appropriate for studying Vietnam veterans.

Cohort Studies

Cohort studies require defining a population of interest, selecting study subjects who will be representative of the larger group, and choosing whether it is more appropriate (or feasible) to study the group's cumulative health experience up to the time of the study (a retrospective approach) or to follow the group into the future to observe changes in their health status (a prospective approach).

One challenge for a cohort study is identifying the members of a population of interest from which a study sample can be selected. A complete roster, or even a representative sample, of U.S. veterans who served in Vietnam is not readily available to researchers outside VA. An alternative approach would be to make use of all or a subsample of a group of Vietnam veterans selected for a previous study. Oversampling those who were closer to herbicide spraying may improve statistical power.

Obtaining information on potential confounding variables (e.g., tobacco, alcohol, or drug use) will be important. It may be possible to control confounding indirectly to some degree by controlling for military rank or other socioeconomic factors or else by stratifying or restricting the analyses on the basis of other related variables, such as the level of potential combat experience. With a retrospective cohort approach it may be difficult to obtain accurate information on confounders, particularly for those study subjects who are deceased. In a prospective cohort study, Vietnam veterans who are alive today would be interviewed to obtain information on potential confounding factors and then followed to determine their subsequent incidence of or mortality from diseases of interest.

Other tradeoffs between retrospective and prospective approaches should also be considered. A prospective cohort study will take many years to accrue a sufficient number of cases for a meaningful analysis. It will probably be considerably more expensive than a retrospective study because of the need to identify and monitor large populations over extended periods into the future. Even a retrospective study, though likely to be less expensive than a prospective study, will still be expensive because of the need to conduct extensive manual searching to obtain the necessary troop assignment information for linkage with the Stellman team's exposure assessment model.

Because of the costs that are likely to be associated with conducting an entirely new cohort study, the most practical approach may be to start with study groups that have already been assembled. Some of the previously studied populations are described later in this chapter.

Case-Control Studies

An alternative to conducting cohort studies would be to use a case-control approach. Case-control studies involve selecting cases of a particular disease (e.g., specific cancers, diabetes, a neurologic disease) as well as a set of controls who are representative of the population from which the cases developed. This is the strategy being followed by Dr. Stellman (2007c) in a study of ALS and by Dr. Han Kang and colleagues at VA in a study of soft tissue sarcoma (VA, 2007). The primary advantage of a case-control approach over a cohort study is that the cost of obtaining information on study subjects is much lower because the size of the study population is much smaller.

Because of the expense involved in obtaining data on study subjects' location histories and lifestyle factors (e.g., tobacco, alcohol, and drug use), a case-control approach may be the most cost-effective design for studying Vietnam veterans. Among case-control studies, those in which cases and controls are sampled from a defined cohort would be optimal. The controls can be randomly selected either from those subjects at risk at the beginning of the cohort study (generally referred to as a case-cohort design) or from those subjects at risk of developing the disease at the time each case occurred (generally referred to as a nested case-control study).

POTENTIAL STUDY POPULATIONS

Using existing study populations and databases for an epidemiologic investigation of Vietnam veterans is desirable because of the expense and logistical difficulties in constructing a study database. The committee is aware of the following potential study populations that should be considered for studies using the Stellman team's model.

VA Study Populations and Registries

One source of frustration for researchers in the years following the Vietnam War was the lack of a comprehensive list of U.S. military personnel who had served in Vietnam. In response to an IOM (1994) recommendation, DoD and VA worked together to compile of list of those who served in Vietnam, using three data sources: the VA Beneficiary Identification and Record Locator Subsystem (BIRLS), DoD personnel files and post-service files, and state rosters of recipients of Vietnam service bonuses (Kang, 2007a). Completed in 1996, the roster includes more than 3 million veterans, of whom 50 percent are identified as having served in the Army, 17 percent in the Air Force, 13 percent in the Marine Corps, 8 percent in the Navy, 0.1 percent in the Coast Guard, and 12 percent with no branch of service identified.

The contribution that this roster could make to studies of Vietnam veterans needs further evaluation, but the roster could prove a useful starting point if access issues can be overcome. Its large size makes it particularly attractive as a potential sampling frame for conducting a cohort study, but the database does not have complete information for all records. For example, only 64 percent of the records include both start and end dates of military service (Kang, 2007b). Furthermore, the database does not include the dates for each veteran's arrival in and departure from the Vietnam theater of operations. If the roster were approached without a means of selecting for members of specific units for which location histories can be determined on a group basis, the challenge of developing the location information and assigning exposures to large numbers of individuals using the Stellman team's exposure model would be considerable. One promising approach would be to conduct follow-up on the entire cohort and then to perform nested case-control studies for outcomes of a priori interest or for any outcomes that are found to be in excess in the cohort. This approach, if feasible, would minimize the amount of work involved in obtaining the location information and other information needed for estimating exposures.

As noted in Chapter 4, VA also has electronic databases that include information on mortality and inpatient and outpatient treatment as well as special registries for veterans with conditions such as ALS and multiple sclerosis. These resources have been used in the past for case-control studies of Vietnam veterans. For example, Dalager et al. (1991) examined the association between non-Hodgkin's lymphoma (NHL) and service in Vietnam. The study included 201 Vietnam-era veterans with NHL and 358 with diagnoses other than any form of malignant lymphoma, all of whom were identified using the VA Patient Treatment File (PTF). The investigators were able to establish whether the study subjects had served in Vietnam and to gather information on dates of service, military occupational specialty codes, and unit identifications for each assignment by reviewing military service records at the National Personnel Records Center in St. Louis. VA has also carried out case-control studies for soft-tissue sarcoma (Kang et al., 1986), Hodgkin's disease (Dalager et al., 1995), lung cancer (Mahan et al., 1997), and testicular cancer (Bullman et al., 1994). An important limitation of this approach is that it will be based only on the population of veterans who receive medical care from VA.

VA has also carried out mortality studies of Vietnam veterans who served in the Army or Marine Corps (e.g., Breslin et al., 1988; Watanabe and Kang, 1995, 1996). The most recent of these studies included approximately 33,800 deceased veterans who had served in Vietnam. The data abstracted from their military personnel records included their dates of Vietnam service, principal duty, and unit addresses. As noted below, VA researchers are planning to explore application of the Stellman team's model to these study populations (VA, 2007).

In addition, VA maintains the Agent Orange Registry, which includes about 409,000 Vietnam veterans (Kang, 2007a). This registry is composed of individuals who volunteered for a physical examination because of their concerns regarding herbicide exposure. Its membership may have a high proportion of those veterans who were proximal to spraying, potentially making it a useful source of somewhat more highly exposed study subjects. However, the registry also has the potential to selectively include not only those who were proximal to spraying but also those who suffered health problems perceived as being associated with herbicide exposure. If so, this combination would introduce a bias into any study of the health effects associated with herbicide exposure that was performed on a population selected from this registry.

The CDC Agent Orange Study

In the 1980s, the Centers for Disease Control and Prevention (CDC) initiated work on three studies of Vietnam veterans, one of which was intended to focus on the health effects of Agent Orange exposure. The exposure study was planned to include approximately 17,000 soldiers from 65 Army combat battalions that served in III Corps during 1967–1968 (CDC, 1985). Selection criteria for individual study subjects included the following: (1) draftees and single-term enlistees, (2) pay grades E1 through E5, (3) only one tour of duty in Vietnam, and (4) at least 6 months served in a single unit. Plans for the study were abandoned after a related CDC validation study found that serum levels of TCDD in Vietnam veterans were not significantly different from those of veterans who did not serve in Vietnam and bore no relationship to the proximity-based exposure measures used in the study (CDC, 1988).

The unit location records collected for the Agent Orange Exposure study were later located by the Stellman team and have been further cleaned and checked (Stellman and Stellman, 2003), making them a potentially useful resource for studies of the health effects of herbicide exposure. Other potential resources are public-use data files constructed by CDC in conjunction with its validation study as well as a separate Vietnam Experience Study (Barrett, 2007). CDC also holds additional data files related to these studies that are protected by confidentiality agreements.

One major limitation of the CDC groups as potential study populations is that the soldiers with greater exposure opportunity may have been eliminated from the studies because of the requirement that eligible subjects have only one tour of duty in Vietnam. Another concern is that the study populations may not be large enough to permit the detection of risk for rarer health effects, such as soft tissue sarcomas or NHL.

Units Identified as More Highly Exposed Based on the Stellman Team's Exposure Assessment Model

Other potential targets for study that warrant consideration are members of military units for which location histories have already been tracked and for which the exposure assessment model suggests the likelihood of higher exposure compared with other units. In other words, units with high EOI values could be selected for further investigation. Alternatively, groups with the potential for greater herbicide exposure could be identified by examining the map of sprayed areas in conjunction with approximately known locations of military units.

The cancelled CDC study of the 1980s used the approach of selecting units that had served in areas of heavy spraying. However, future researchers who take a similar approach may want to include study participants with more than one tour of duty and take full advantage of the knowledge gained by the Stellman team in their efforts to characterize exposures by service unit. Even with unit location histories, researchers will still need to compile full unit assignment histories for individual subjects and ascertain their health experience.

The committee notes that the Air Force Ranch Hand personnel and Army Chemical Corps personnel are two groups of veterans that are not suitable study populations when the Stellman team's model is to be used, even though their exposures to herbicides are likely to be among the highest of all veterans. Most of their herbicide exposures were a direct result of duties that required handling or applying herbicides. By contrast, the model is designed to assess the exposure opportunity that would result from unintended proximity to herbicide spraying.

Australian and Korean Veterans of Vietnam

Approximately 59,200 Australian men have been identified as veterans of military service in Vietnam (Wilson et al., 2005b), and numerous studies have been made of the morbidity and mortality of Australian veterans (e.g., see list in Wilson and Horsley, 2003). A third round of retrospective cohort studies commissioned by the Australian government was completed in 2005 (Wilson et al., 2005a,b,c).

Some studies of Australian veterans of the Vietnam War have relied on comparisons with the general Australian population to assess health risks, with the most recent reports showing elevated risks of certain cancers (e.g., lung and prostate) and liver disease (Wilson et al., 2005b,c). For many other conditions, veterans have lower risks than the general population. In studies specifically of conscripted veterans, comparisons have been made between those who served in Vietnam (approximately 19,200 men) and those who did not (24,700 men) (e.g., Fett et al., 1987; Crane et al., 1997; Wilson et al., 2005a). The most recent of these studies found that Vietnam veterans had significantly higher incidence and mortality rates of lung and pancreatic cancers and a higher incidence of head and neck cancer (Wilson et al., 2005a).

The effects of herbicide exposure have been a concern among Australian veterans, and, as with many studies of U.S. veterans, service in Vietnam has often constituted the exposure criterion in Australian studies. Thus Australian veterans would seem to present another opportunity for application of the Stellman team's exposure assessment model. A searchable roster of these veterans has been compiled and is accessible through the Internet (http://www.vietnamroll.gov.au/). In communications with Dr. Keith Horsley (2007a,b) of the Australian Institute of Health and Welfare, the committee also learned that records of ground troop locations are poor for land-based Australian Navy and Air Force personnel and generally good for most Australian Army units (the Australian Task Force). According to Dr. Horsley, location information for the Task Force, roughly 38,000 men, is frequently available down to the section level of nine people. The Australian military records are in paper form and stored in the archives of the Australian Department of Defense (Horsley, 2007a). Reconstructing troop locations for Australian service members would seem to pose some of the same challenges as for U.S. troops. The committee did not explore access issues for these records but can see application of the exposure assessment model as a reasonable possibility.

Approximately 320,000 South Korean soldiers also participated in the Vietnam War, and more than 92,000 soldiers have reported having health problems related to Agent Orange exposure (Kim et al., 2003). A research group conducted a study of morbidity and mortality of Korean soldiers using EOI values from the Stellman team's model (Yonsei Medical Institution, 2006).[5] To the best of the committee's knowledge, this is the only completed analysis to date that has used the current version of the Stellman team's model. Complete information on study methods and findings was not available to the committee at the time this report was written, but the approach is of particular interest as an example of the application of the exposure assessment model. As details become available, the design and results of this study may be of use to other researchers planning to apply the model.

---

[5]Personal communication, S.-W. Yi, Kwandong University, August 17, 2007.

Residents of Vietnam

The Stellman team's model may also be of use in estimating potential herbicide exposures and studying health outcomes in Vietnamese soldiers and civilians. With the possible exception of the U.S. Air Force personnel participating in Operation Ranch Hand and the Army Chemical Corps, it is likely that the Vietnamese population experienced higher levels of exposure than did U.S. troops because of the greater opportunity of the Vietnamese to be exposed through multiple routes, including inhalation, ingestion of local food and water, and dermal contact with soil and sediments in sprayed areas. Although the possibility of applying the Stellman team's model to studies of the Vietnamese is of interest and potentially informative about the health effects of herbicides, the committee saw such studies as contributing only indirectly to a better understanding of the health of U.S. veterans, which was the focus of its charge.

Committee Observations

The committee sees the potential for researchers to pursue studies in a variety of Vietnam veteran populations, while noting that each population presents different trade-offs in terms of magnitude of effort, the availability of data on locations of service in Vietnam, representation of those more likely to have been exposed, and access to data on health outcomes. Researchers will need to direct their efforts based on the particulars of their research questions and on available resources. The committee believes that the most promising studies are either those that use groups where higher exposure to herbicides appears likely based on analysis of existing unit or troop movement information, or case-control studies nested in large cohorts already assembled, possibly including the VA roster of 3 million Vietnam veterans.

ONGOING VA WORK TO APPLY THE EXPOSURE ASSESSMENT MODEL

Dr. Han Kang and colleagues at VA have several projects under way to explore use of the Stellman team's model (VA, 2007). The work "aims to evaluate the validity and utility of this model . . . using the databases already collected from previous health studies on Vietnam veterans." They have described three specific areas of inquiry:

1. Does the model generate internally consistent index exposure scores that are consistent with variation in military mission? To test this, five military units stationed in Vietnam during the height of Agent Orange

spraying in 1968 will be tracked for geographic location in Vietnam for one year, using the databases already collected by Dr. Stellman and her team.

2. Does the model demonstrate a positive association between the index exposure scores and the prevalence or incidence of health outcomes that are considered truly associated with herbicides, such as soft tissue sarcoma, non-Hodgkin's lymphoma, and Hodgkin's disease? To test this, veteran study subjects from three existing case-control study databases and three Vietnam veterans' mortality study databases will be used. Geographic locations and time of service in Vietnam will be tracked for the cancer cases and the controls and then applied to the model.

3. Does application of the model to existing epidemiologic study databases generate additional information on the health effects of exposure to herbicide in Vietnam beyond what is already known? How much time and resources are required to conduct a health study of Vietnam veterans using the model? The model will be applied to three existing databases: the Agent Orange Registry of 409,000 Vietnam veterans, Marine Corps Vietnam Veterans, and Women Vietnam Veterans.

When Dr. Kang and his colleagues met with the committee in spring 2007, they reported that efforts were under way to construct location histories for the veterans who would be included in the reanalyses. Calculation of exposure metrics using the Stellman team's model had not yet begun.

The committee sees the value of VA's work in investigating the feasibility of obtaining the needed model inputs and generating exposure scores. Because of its unique insights into military records and databases, the VA research group has the potential for achieving success that can be documented and shared with other researchers beyond VA. Completion of this work should thus prove worthwhile and informative for methodologic purposes in addition to generating epidemiologic findings that relate estimated exposure opportunity to particular health outcomes.

Nevertheless, as has previously been observed (IOM, 2003), such studies are of limited value in moving toward the stated goal of validating the model. If positive, these studies would lend support to the model's potential use. If the results are negative, though, the findings will be difficult to interpret. They cannot disprove the value of the proximity model because the levels of exposure may be lower than would cause adverse health effects or because the study's power may be insufficient to address the question adequately.

Although the work that the VA researchers are conducting will make an important contribution, its scope falls short of the complete array of work that the committee believes would be appropriate. The committee understands that not all the efforts it proposes can be undertaken at once, but it does have some specific concerns. In the morbidity studies that are to be revisited, the range of health outcomes is limited, the ascertainment of those health outcomes ended for the most recent of the studies in 1985,[6] and the health data are limited to events identified among veterans who participated in the VA health care system. There do not appear to be plans to conduct sensitivity analyses or explore ways in which the model might be extended. In addition, there is no indication of plans to create a resource that other investigators, including those outside VA, could expand upon. For these reasons, the committee sees the VA work as insufficient by itself to constitute the best use of the exposure assessment model.

CONTRIBUTION TO THE ONGOING IOM REVIEWS OF THE ASSOCIATION BETWEEN HERBICIDE EXPOSURE AND HEALTH OUTCOMES

The biennial reviews carried out by IOM committees to examine potential associations between herbicide exposure and health effects have had to rely in large measure on studies in populations other than Vietnam veterans to reach conclusions regarding the strength of such associations. Application of the herbicide exposure assessment model in epidemiologic studies of Vietnam veterans has the potential to contribute to the body of work that future committees can evaluate. No single study should be expected to provide definitive evidence, but results derived from studies of the population of interest will be a welcome addition. The committee reiterates, however, that because of the potential for exposure misclassification and concerns about statistical power, studies of Vietnam veterans that make use of the proximity-based exposure surrogates must always be viewed as informative rather than definitive.

CONCLUSIONS

The committee reached the following specific conclusions regarding the use of the Stellman team's herbicide exposure assessment model in epidemiologic studies:

1. Epidemiologic studies of health outcomes among Vietnam veterans that use the exposure opportunity index are capable of characterizing the health of veterans in relation to their proximity to herbicide spraying. Such studies would provide an improvement in evaluating potential effects of herbicide exposure compared to studies based on Vietnam service in gen-

---

[6]Case ascertainment for the case-control studies carried out by VA extended to the following years: NHL, 1985 (Dalager et al., 1991); Hodgkin's disease, 1985 (Dalager et al., 1995); and soft tissue sarcoma, 1983 (Kang et al., 1986).

eral. This improvement may permit observation of associations between herbicide exposure and health effects in the Vietnam veteran population that were not identifiable in previous studies.

2. The ongoing efforts by the VA investigators to apply the model in existing case-control study populations are useful for characterizing the logistical challenges and the magnitude of effort needed to apply the model, but they are limited and insufficiently accessible to future researchers and the broader research community and so do not constitute, in isolation, the best use of the exposure assessment model.

3. The most promising study designs for applications of the model would be (1) to selectively sample units based on exposure potential, gathering relevant information from unit records, individual service records, and sources of individual health outcomes data; or (2) to build on large cohorts already assembled and pursue nested case-control studies of outcomes of interest with linkage to units, unit locations, and exposure potential.

4. Efforts to validate the model solely by examining health outcomes believed to be related to herbicide exposure are of limited value. If positive, such studies would add support to the model's potential value, but, if negative, the model's value would not be disproved because the levels of exposure may be lower than would cause adverse health effects or the study's power may be insufficient to address the question adequately.

RECOMMENDATIONS

The committee's conclusions from its consideration of the Stellman team's herbicide exposure assessment model led it to make the following recommendations:

1. **VA should sponsor epidemiologic studies of Vietnam veterans that take into account the criteria below regarding the appropriate characteristics of informative research on herbicide exposure and health outcomes in this population. VA should draw on the criteria as the basis for developing a request for proposals.**

   Specifically, to make the best use of the exposure assessment model, epidemiologic studies of Vietnam veterans should have the following characteristics:

   a. The study population should be broadly representative of Vietnam veterans, with care taken to include sufficient numbers of study participants with relatively higher exposure.
   b. A broad range of health outcomes should be considered, not just those that are suspected of being related to herbicide expo-

sure. Where feasible, morbidity should be studied in addition to mortality.
c. The health data should be as complete and up-to-date as possible.
d. The study should have sufficient statistical power to address the range of health outcomes of concern.
e. To isolate the effects of herbicide exposure, potential confounding factors need to be carefully addressed in the study design or the analytic approach.
f. Analyses should be conducted to evaluate how sensitive the estimated associations between exposure opportunity and health outcomes are to the uncertainty in the exposure opportunity metrics and to varying approaches to estimating herbicide exposure, possibly including alternative approaches to exposure assignment as discussed in Chapter 3.
g. Opportunities to conduct research using the exposure assessment model should be open to investigators beyond the VA system to allow for the benefits of engaging the broader research community and to enhance public acceptance and credibility.

2. In support of the recommended epidemiologic studies, VA should work with DoD and NARA to

- facilitate health research uses of military records that are subject to access barriers arising from privacy laws, and
- arrange for assistance from DoD and NARA staff with appropriate expertise to aid researchers in the location and interpretation of military records for health research uses.

REFERENCES

Barrett, D. H. 2007. *Letter to L. Joellenbeck, with accompanying materials.* Atlanta, GA, June 22.

Breslin, P., H. K. Kang, Y. Lee, V. Burt, and B. Shepard. 1988. Proportionate mortality study of US Army and US Marine Corps veterans of the Vietnam War. *Journal of Occupational Medicine* 30(5):412–419.

Bullman, T. A., K. K. Watanabe, and H. K. Kang. 1994. Risk of testicular cancer associated with surrogate measures of Agent Orange exposure among Vietnam veterans on the Agent Orange Registry. *Annals of Epidemiology* 4:11–16.

CDC (Centers for Disease Control and Prevention). 1985. *Exposure assessment for the Agent Orange study.* Interim Report Number 2. Typescript.

CDC. 1988. Serum 2,3,7,8-tetrachlorodibenzo-*p*-dioxin levels in U.S. Army Vietnam-era veterans. The Centers for Disease Control Veterans Health Studies. *Journal of the American Medical Association* 260(9):1249–1254.

CDC. 1989. *Comparison of serum levels of 2,3,7,8-tetrachlorodibenzo-p-dioxin with indirect estimates of Agent Orange exposure among Vietnam veterans: Final report.* Atlanta, GA: Agent Orange Projects, Center for Environmental Health and Injury Control.

Crane, P. J., D. L. Barnard, K. W. Horsley, M. A. Adena. 1997. *Mortality of national service Vietnam veterans: A report of the 1996 retrospective cohort study of Australian Vietnam veterans.* Canberra, Australia: Department of Veterans' Affairs.

Dalager, N. A., H. K. Kang, V. L. Burt, and L. Weatherbee. 1991. Non-Hodgkin's lymphoma among Vietnam veterans. *Journal of Occupational Medicine* 33(7):774–779.

Dalager, N. A., H. K. Kang, V. L. Burt, and L. Weatherbee. 1995. Hodgkin's disease and Vietnam service. *Annals of Epidemiology* 5(5):400–406.

Dominici, F., S. L. Zeger, and J. M. Samet. 2000. A measurement error model for time-series studies of air pollution and mortality. *Biostatistics* 1(2):157–175.

Dwernychuk, L. W. 2005. Dioxin hot spots in Vietnam. *Chemosphere* 60:998–999.

Dwernychuk, L. W., H. D. Cau, C. T. Hatfield, T. G. Boivin, T. M. Hung, P. T. Dung, and N. D. Thai. 2002. Dioxin reservoirs in southern Viet Nam—A legacy of Agent Orange. *Chemosphere* 47(2):117–137.

Fett, M. J., J. R. Nairn, D. M. Cobbin, and M. A. Adena. 1987. Mortality among Australian conscripts of the Vietnam conflict era. II. Causes of death. *American Journal of Epidemiology* 125:878–884.

Flegal, K. M., C. Brownie, and J. D. Haas. 1986. The effects of exposure misclassification on estimates of relative risk. *American Journal of Epidemiology* 123(4):736–751.

Greenland, S. 2000. Principles of multilevel modeling. *International Journal of Epidemiology* 29:158–167.

Hatfield Consultants and Office of the National Steering Committee 33, MNRE (Ministry of Natural Resources and Environment, Vietnam). 2007. *Assessment of dioxin contamination in the environment and human population in the vicinity of Da Nang Airbase, Viet Nam: Final report.* West Vancouver, British Columbia, Canada.

Horsley, K. 2007a. *Re: Inquiry regarding Australian veterans and Agent Orange studies.* E-mail to L. Joellenbeck, June 4.

Horsley, K. 2007b. *Re: Inquiry regarding Australian veterans and Agent Orange studies.* E-mail to L. Joellenbeck, June 28.

IOM (Institute of Medicine). 1994. *Veterans and Agent Orange: Health effects of herbicides used in Vietnam.* Washington, DC: National Academy Press.

IOM. 2003. *Characterizing exposure of veterans to Agent Orange and other herbicides used in Vietnam: Interim findings and recommendations.* Washington, DC: The National Academies Press.

IOM. 2007. *Veterans and Agent Orange: Update 2006.* Washington, DC: The National Academies Press.

Kang, H. K. 2007a. *Data resources within VA for an epidemiological study of Vietnam veterans.* PowerPoint presentation to the IOM Committee on Making Best Use of the Agent Orange Reconstruction Model, Meeting 2, April 30–May 1, Washington, DC.

Kang, H. K. 2007b. *Vietnam roster veterans: Demographic/military service characteristics.* Unpublished document submitted to the IOM Committee on Making the Best Use of the Agent Orange Reconstruction Model, July 11.

Kang, H. K., L. Weatherbee, P. Breslin, Y. Lee, and B. Shepard. 1986. Soft tissue sarcomas and military service in Vietnam: A case comparison group analysis of hospital patients. *Journal of Occupational and Environmental Medicine* 28(12):1215–1218.

Kim, H. A., E. M. Kim, Y. C. Park, J. Y. Yu, S. K. Hong, S. H. Jeon, K. L. Park, S. J. Hur, and Y. Heo. 2003. Immunotoxicological effects of Agent Orange exposure to the Vietnam War Korean veterans. *Industrial Health* 41:158–166.

Mahan, C. M., T. A. Bullman, and H. K. Kang. 1997. A case-control study of lung cancer among Vietnam veterans. *Journal of Occupational and Environmental Medicine* 39(8):740–747.

McFall, M. E., M. E. Mackay, and D. M. Donovan. 1992. Combat-related posttraumatic stress disorder and severity of substance abuse in Vietnam veterans. *Journal of Studies on Alcohol* 53(4):357–363.

Michalek, J. E., S. P. Caudill, and R. C. Tripathi. 1996. Pharmacokinetics of TCDD in veterans of Operation Ranch Hand: 10-year follow-up. *Journal of Toxicology and Environmental Health* 47:209–220.

Mocarelli, P., L. L. Needham, A. Marocchi, D. G. Patterson, Jr., P. Brambilla, P. M. Gerthoux, L. Meazza, and V. Carreri. 1991. Serum concentrations of 2,3,7,8-tetrachlorodibenzo-*p*-dioxin and test results from selected residents of Seveso, Italy. *Journal of Toxicology and Environmental Health* 32:357–366.

Peng, R. D., F. Dominici, and S. L. Zeger. 2006. Reproducible epidemiologic research. *American Journal of Epidemiology* 163(9):783–789.

Pirkle, J. L., and V. N. Houk. 1992. Use of epidemiologic studies to assess human risk from exposure to 2,3,7,8-tetrachlorodibenzo-*p*-dioxin. *Chemosphere* 25(7–10):1109–1115.

Stayner, L., M. Vrijheid, E. Cardis, D. O. Stram, I. Deltour, S. J. Gilbert, and G. Howe. 2007. A Monte Carlo maximum likelihood method for estimating uncertainty arising from shared errors in exposures in epidemiological studies of nuclear workers. *Radiation Research* 168(6):757–763.

Stellman, J. M. 2007a. *A data resource for the health and environmental consequences of the Vietnam War.* Unpublished document submitted to the IOM Committee on Making the Best Use of the Agent Orange Reconstruction Model, July 31.

Stellman, J. M. 2007b. *Responses to IOM 091407.* Unpublished document submitted to the IOM Committee on Making the Best Use of the Agent Orange Reconstruction Model, September 14.

Stellman, J. M. 2007c. *Separate modeling and reconstruction issues.* PowerPoint presentation to the IOM Committee on Making Best Use of the Agent Orange Reconstruction Model, Meeting 3, June 13–14, Washington, DC.

Stellman, J. M., and S. D. Stellman. 2003. *Contractor's final report: Characterizing exposure of veterans to Agent Orange and other herbicides in Vietnam.* Submitted to the National Academy of Sciences, Institute of Medicine, in fulfillment of Subcontract VA-5124-98-0019, June 30, 2003.

Sweeney, M. H., G. M. Calvert, G. A. Egeland, M. A. Fingerhut, W. E. Halperin, and L. A. Piacitelli. 1997–1998. Review and update of the results of the NIOSH medical study of workers exposed to chemicals contaminated with 2,3,7,8-tetrachlorodibenzodioxin. *Teratogenesis, Carcinogenesis, and Mutagenesis* 17(4–5):241–247.

VA (U.S. Department of Veterans Affairs). 2007. *Evaluation of Dr. Stellman's herbicide exposure reconstruction model.* http://www.va.gov/wriisc-dc/research/studies_ongoing.asp#Stellman (accessed February 22, 2007).

Watanabe, K. K., and H. K. Kang. 1995. Military service in Vietnam and the risk of death from trauma and selected cancers. *Annals of Epidemiology* 5:407–412.

Watanabe, K. K., and H. K. Kang. 1996. Mortality patterns among Vietnam veterans. *Journal of Occupational and Environmental Medicine* 38(3):272–278.

Wilson, E. J., and K. W. A. Horsley. 2003. Health effects of Vietnam service. *ADF Health* 4:59–65.

Wilson, E. J., K. W. Horsley, and R. van der Hoek. 2005a. *Australian National Service Vietnam Veterans Mortality and Cancer Incidence Study 2005.* Canberra, Australia: Department of Veterans' Affairs.

Wilson, E. J., K. W. Horsley, and R. van der Hoek. 2005b. *Australian Vietnam Veterans Mortality Study 2005*. Canberra, Australia: Department of Veterans' Affairs.

Wilson, E. J., K. W. Horsley, and R. van der Hoek. 2005c. *Cancer Incidence in Australian Vietnam Veterans Study 2005*. Canberra, Australia: Department of Veterans' Affairs.

Yonsei Medical Institution. 2006. [*Final report: Dynamic study for defoliant (Agent Orange) damages.*] Report to the Ministry of Patriots and Veterans Affairs, Republic of Korea.

Appendix A

Agendas for Information-Gathering Meetings

Meeting 1
March 8–9, 2007

The Keck Center of the National Academies
500 Fifth Street, N.W.
Washington, DC

Thursday, March 8, 2007

10:00 a.m. Introductory Remarks
David Savitz, Ph.D.
Chair, Committee on Making Best Use of the Agent Orange Exposure Reconstruction Model

Introductions by committee members and meeting attendees

10:15 a.m. Study Context and Goals, Sponsor Perspective
Mark Brown, Ph.D.
Director, Environmental Agents Service
Veterans Health Administration, Department of Veterans Affairs

An Introduction to VA Data Resources Relevant to Use of the Exposure Model

Discussion

11:00 a.m.   An Overview of the Agent Orange Exposure Reconstruction Model
Jeanne Mager Stellman, Ph.D.
Steven Stellman, Ph.D., M.P.H.
Mailman School of Public Health, Columbia University

Discussion

12:30 p.m.   Working lunch in meeting room

1:15 p.m.   Additional discussion of the exposure assessment model as needed

1:45 p.m.   The Work of the Joint Services Records Research Center
Donald Hakenson
Director, Joint Services Records Research Center

Discussion

2:15 p.m.   General discussion

3:00 p.m.   Opportunity for public comment

4:00 p.m.   Adjourn open session

Meeting 2
April 30–May 1, 2007

The Keck Center of the National Academies
500 Fifth Street, N.W.
Washington, DC

Monday, April 30, 2007

1:30 p.m.   Introductory Remarks
David Savitz, Ph.D.
Chair, Committee on Making Best Use of the Agent Orange Exposure Reconstruction Model

Introductions by committee members and meeting attendees

APPENDIX A   115

1:45 p.m.   VA Data Resources Relevant to Use of the Agent Orange
               Exposure Model
               Han Kang, Ph.D.
               Director, Environmental Epidemiology Service
               Director, War-Related Injury and Illness Study Center
               Department of Veterans Affairs

               Discussion

2:30 p.m.   Review of the CDC Agent Orange Exposure Index and
               Validation Study
               Thomas H. Sinks, Ph.D.
               *Deputy Director, National Center for Environmental
               Health/ATSDR*
               Centers for Disease Control and Prevention

               Discussion

3:15 p.m.   Accessing Military Unit Records at the College Park Archives
               Richard Boylan
               National Archives and Records Administration

               Discussion

3:45 p.m.   Accessing Service Member Personnel Records via the IOM
               Medical Follow-up Agency
               William Page, Ph.D., and Harriet Crawford, B.S.
               Institute of Medicine Medical Follow-up Agency

               Discussion

4:15 p.m.   General discussion

4:30 p.m.   Adjourn open session

               Tuesday, May 1, 2007

8:30 a.m.   Introductory Remarks
               David Savitz, Ph.D.
               *Chair, Committee on Making Best Use of the Agent Orange
               Exposure Reconstruction Model*

8:45 a.m.	Environmental Fate of TCDD: Relationships to Human Exposure in Vietnam *Alvin L. Young, Ph.D.* *Visiting Professor, Institute for Science and Public Policy* *The University of Oklahoma* *John P. Giesy, Ph.D.* *Canada Research Chair in Environmental Toxicology* *University of Saskatchewan* Discussion
9:30 a.m.	Michigan's Dioxin Exposure Study: Findings of Interest for Agent Orange Exposure Assessment *David H. Garabrant, M.D., M.P.H.* *Professor, Occupational Medicine and Epidemiology* *The University of Michigan School of Public Health* Discussion
10:00 a.m.	Perspectives on Agent Orange Exposure Reconstruction in Vietnam *Marie Haring Sweeney, Ph.D., M.P.H.* *Chief, Surveillance Branch* *Division of Surveillance, Hazard Evaluations & Field Studies* *National Institute for Occupational Safety and Health* Discussion
10:45 a.m.	Points to Consider When Evaluating the Stellman Model *John H. Ross, Ph.D., DABT* *Director, Environmental Sciences* *Infoscientific.com, Inc.* *Michael E. Ginevan, Ph.D.* *M.E. Ginevan & Associates* Discussion
11:15 a.m.	General discussion
11:45 a.m.	Adjourn open session

APPENDIX A   *117*

Meeting 3
June 13–14, 2007

The Keck Center of the National Academies
500 Fifth Street, N.W.
Washington, DC

Wednesday, June 13, 2007

1:30 p.m.	Introductory Remarks *David A. Savitz, Ph.D.* *Chair, Committee on Making Best Use of the Agent Orange Exposure Reconstruction Model* Introductions by committee members and meeting attendees
1:35 p.m.	Demonstration of the Agent Orange Exposure Reconstruction Model and Advice on Tracking Units *Jeanne Mager Stellman, Ph.D.* *Steven Stellman, Ph.D., M.P.H.* *Mailman School of Public Health, Columbia University* Discussion
2:40 p.m.	Adjourn open session

Thursday, June 14, 2007

8:30 a.m.	Introductory Remarks *David A. Savitz, Ph.D.* *Chair, Committee on Making Best Use of the Agent Orange Exposure Reconstruction Model*
8:35 a.m.	Perspectives from the IOM Committee on the Assessment of Wartime Exposure to Herbicides in Vietnam *David J. Tollerud, M.D., M.P.H.* *Professor and Chair* *Department of Environmental & Occupational Health Sciences* *University of Louisville, School of Public Health & Information Sciences*

Discussion

10:00 a.m.   Adjourn open session

Appendix B

Exposure Measures in Studies of U.S. Vietnam Veterans

TABLE B-1 Exposure Measures in Studies of U.S. Vietnam Veterans

Reference	Design	Description	Sources of Exposure Data	Exposure Measures
CDC Studies				
Erickson et al., 1984a,b	Case-control	CDC Birth Defects Study Birth defect cases and normal controls born in the Atlanta, GA, area, 1968–1980	Telephone interview Military records	Veteran (ever served in U.S. military) Vietnam service before conception of case/control offspring EOI (values 1–5): scores assigned on the basis of reviews by Army experts of duties, dates, and places of service in Vietnam; separate scores for information from (1) interviews and (2) review of military records Self-reports of Agent Orange exposure
Boyle et al., 1987; CDC, 1987	Retrospective cohort	CDC Vietnam Experience Study: Mortality in Vietnam and Vietnam-era veterans	Military records	Army service in Vietnam between 1965 and 1971
CDC, 1988 a,b,c; 1989	Cohort	CDC Vietnam Experience Study: Psychosocial, physical health, and reproductive outcomes	Military records Telephone interview	Army service in Vietnam between 1965 and 1971 Self-reported exposures
CDC, 1988d	Cohort pilot	CDC Agent Orange Validation Study Army Vietnam veterans and Vietnam-era controls	Military records Self-report through structured interview	Five scores based on military records; two scores based on information from self-report The scoring methods based on information from military records reflected different assumptions about TCDD half-life and about completeness of data on troop and herbicide spray locations

Study	Design	Population/Outcome	Data Source	Exposure Assessment
CDC, 1990 a,b,c,d	Case-control	Selected Cancer Studies: Studies of NHL, HD, STS, nasal carcinoma, nasopharyngeal carcinoma, liver cancer	Telephone interview, supplemented by review of military records; Classification of unit mission by U.S. Army ESG	Two other scores were based on information from the structured interview (self-report): number of days of direct exposure to herbicides during military service; and number of days of indirect exposure to herbicides during military service Self-reported Vietnam service (in sensitivity analyses, service in Vietnam distinguished from service off the coast) Considered branch of service, unit, location in Vietnam, job duties, tour of duty, rank, perceived exposure to herbicides Non-Vietnam occupational exposure to phenoxy herbicides
O'Brien et al., 1991	Cohort	NHL cases identified within Vietnam Experience Study cohort	Military records; Interview	Vietnam service, noting region of service and military occupation
Decouflé et al., 1992	Cohort	Vietnam Experience Study Relationship of self-reported health to self-reported exposure to herbicides and combat among Army veterans	Military records; Telephone questionnaire	Herbicide exposure index reflecting four categories of increasing intensity of exposure based on self-report
Boehmer et al., 2004	Cohort	Mortality update of Vietnam Experience Study cohort	Military records	Entered military service 1965–1971, at least one tour of Army service in Vietnam

continued

TABLE B-1 Continued

Reference	Design	Description	Sources of Exposure Data	Exposure Measures
Department of Veterans Affairs Studies				
Kang et al., 1986	Case-control	Hospital-based study of Vietnam and Vietnam-era veterans diagnosed with STS, 1969–1983	Military records	Vietnam service
Burt et al., 1987	Retrospective cohort	NHL mortality among Vietnam and Vietnam-era Army and Marine Corps veterans	Military records	Service as a member of Army or Marine Corps in Vietnam between July 4, 1965, and March 1, 1973
Kang et al., 1987	Case-control	STS cases diagnosed at Armed Forces Institute of Pathology (1975–1980); controls from patient logs of referring pathologists	Military records Telephone interview	Vietnam service in Army or Marine Corps, combat-related military occupation, and broad geographic location of individual's unit at time of service
Breslin et al., 1988	Retrospective cohort	Mortality among Vietnam and Vietnam-era Army and Marine Corps veterans	Military records	Service as a member of Army or Marine Corps in Vietnam between July 4, 1965, and March 1, 1973
True et al., 1988	Cross-sectional	Military service in Vietnam and subsequent posttraumatic stress disorder symptoms	Questionnaire	Exposure to combat in Vietnam

Bullman et al., 1990	Cohort	Mortality in Army Vietnam and Vietnam-era veterans who served in Military Region I	Military records	Service in Military Region I
Farberow et al., 1990	Case-control	Suicide and motor vehicle deaths in Los Angeles County among Vietnam and Vietnam-era Army and Marine Corps veterans	Military records Medical examiner's records Next-of-kin interviews	Vietnam service, combat-related military occupation based on military records; aspects of military experience based on next-of-kin report
Goldberg et al., 1990	Cohort	Posttraumatic stress disorder among monozygotic twin pairs serving in the military during the Vietnam era	Military records Questionnaire	Southeast Asia service
Bullman et al., 1991	Case-control	Combat and other service experience in posttraumatic stress disorder cases and controls selected from the VA Agent Orange Registry	Military records	Vietnam service in a combat-related military occupation, having been wounded in Vietnam, having been awarded medals for combat-related Vietnam service
Dalager et al., 1991	Case-control	Vietnam and Vietnam-era veterans diagnosed with NHL in VA hospitals, 1969–1985	Military records	Branch of service, combat role, service within a specific region in Vietnam, extended service in Vietnam

continued

TABLE B-1 Continued

Reference	Design	Description	Sources of Exposure Data	Exposure Measures
Eisen et al., 1991	Cohort	Health status of monozygotic twin pairs who served in the military during the Vietnam era	Mail survey or telephone interviews	Southeast Asia service
Thomas et al., 1991	Cohort	Mortality in women Vietnam veterans and Vietnam-era veterans deceased 1973–1987	Military records	Vietnam service
Watanabe et al., 1991	Retrospective cohort	Follow-up through 1984 of mortality study by Breslin et al., 1988	Military records	Army or Marine Corps service in Vietnam between July 4, 1965, and March 1, 1973
Bullman et al., 1994	Case-control	Testicular cancer cases and controls identified from VA Agent Orange Registry	Military records	Branch of service, type of duty, corps area, and location of individual's unit in relation to recorded Agent Orange spray tracks
Dalager et al., 1995a	Cohort	Mortality study of women Vietnam veterans and Vietnam-era veterans who died 1965–1992 Update of Thomas et al., 1991	Military records	Vietnam service

Dalager et al., 1995b	Case-control	Vietnam and Vietnam-era veterans diagnosed with Hodgkin's disease in VA hospitals, 1969–1985	Military records	Branch of service, combat role, service within a specific region in Vietnam, extended service in Vietnam
Watanabe and Kang, 1995	Cohort	Mortality study of U.S. Marine Vietnam and Vietnam-era veterans Extension of Breslin et al., 1988, and Watanabe et al, 1991	Military records	Vietnam service
Watanabe and Kang, 1996	Cohort	Mortality study of Army and Marine Corps Vietnam and Vietnam-era veterans who died 1965–1988	Military records	Vietnam service
Mahan et al., 1997	Case-control	Lung cancer cases among Vietnam-era veterans	Military records	Vietnam service Location of service member's unit in relation to areas sprayed with herbicides and time elapsed since spraying
McKinney et al., 1997	Cross-sectional	Smoking patterns among veterans and non-veterans	1987 National Medical Expenditure Survey	Vietnam service
Kang et al., 2000a	Cohort	Self-reported pregnancy outcomes for women Vietnam and Vietnam-era veterans	Military records Structured telephone interview	Vietnam service

continued

TABLE B-1 Continued

Reference	Design	Description	Sources of Exposure Data	Exposure Measures
Kang et al., 2000b	Cohort	Gynecologic cancers among women Vietnam and Vietnam-era veterans	Military records Structured telephone interview	Vietnam service
State Studies				
Greenwald et al., 1984	Case-control	STS cases from New York State Cancer Registry, diagnosed 1962–1980; population controls	Interview of study subjects or next of kin	Self- or proxy report of Vietnam service, exposure to Agent Orange
Newell, 1984	Cross-sectional	Pilot analyses of cytogenetics, sperm evaluation, and immune response in Vietnam veterans from Texas	Military records Questionnaire	Exposure to herbicides based on the amount of herbicide sprayed in the area where the individual served during period of service Reported presence of chloracne
Kogan and Clapp, 1985	Cohort	Mortality study of Massachusetts Vietnam and Vietnam-era veterans, deceased 1972–1983	List of Massachusetts veterans who served between 1958 and 1973 and received a bonus	Vietnam service
Lawrence et al., 1985	Cohort	Mortality study of veterans discharged from service 1971–1973 and deceased in New York through 1980	Military records (Vietnam service indicators in DMDC roster)	Vietnam service

Rellahan, 1985	Cohort	Survey of residents of Oahu, Hawaii, with Vietnam-era military service	Questionnaire	Vietnam service
Wendt, 1985	Descriptive	Survey of Iowa Vietnam and Vietnam-era veterans	Iowa Department of Veterans Affairs records Questionnaire	Self-reported spraying or handling of Agent Orange, or passing through a sprayed area
Anderson et al., 1986	Cohort	Mortality study of Wisconsin Vietnam veterans, Vietnam-era veterans, and non-veterans	Military records	Vietnam service
Goun and Kuller, 1986	Case-control	Mortality from STS, NHL, and other cancers among Pennsylvania male Vietnam veterans	Federal military records Commonwealth of Pennsylvania Department of Military Affairs records	Vietnam service
Holmes et al., 1986	Cohort	Mortality study of West Virginia Vietnam veterans	List of recipients of West Virginia Vietnam-era service bonus	Vietnam service

continued

TABLE B-1 Continued

Reference	Design	Description	Sources of Exposure Data	Exposure Measures
Pollei et al., 1986	Case-control	Chest radiographs of Vietnam veterans in Albuquerque VA Agent Orange registry; compared to Air Force personnel with no Vietnam service	Interviews; some military records	Registry enrollment; self-reported repeated exposure to Agent Orange
Kahn et al., 1988	Pilot exposure study	Herbicide exposure study of Vietnam and Vietnam-era veterans	Self report, validated with examination of military records by U.S. Army ESG	Highly exposed to Agent Orange (by job title and self-report) Adipose tissue and blood serum measurement of TCDD
Kogan and Clapp, 1988	Cohort	Mortality study of Massachusetts Vietnam and Vietnam-era veterans, deceased 1972–1983; focus on cancer mortality	List of Massachusetts veterans who served between 1958 and 1973 and received a bonus	Vietnam service
Levy, 1988	Cross-sectional	PTSD in those with chloracne among a subset of Massachusetts Vietnam bonus recipients	Telephone interview Medical examination	Current diagnosis of chloracne

Reference	Study Design	Study Population	Exposure Assessment
Clapp et al., 1991	Case-control	Cancer cases from Massachusetts Cancer Registry, diagnosed 1982–1988	List of Massachusetts veterans who served between 1958 and 1973 and received a bonus	Vietnam service
Deprez et al., 1991	Descriptive	Health status and reproductive outcomes in Maine Vietnam veterans	Questionnaire	Self-reported exposure to herbicides
Fiedler et al., 1992; Kahn et al., 1992a,b	Cohort	Health outcomes in New Jersey Vietnam and Vietnam-era veterans	Self report, validated with examination of military records by U.S. Army ESG	TCDD in blood; service in units that operated in heavily sprayed areas of Vietnam
Visintainer et al., 1995	Cohort	Mortality study of Michigan Vietnam and Vietnam-era veterans	Michigan bonus list	Vietnam service ("in-country" versus "out-country")
Clapp, 1997	Case-control	Cancer cases from Massachusetts Cancer Registry, diagnosed 1982–1993 Update of Clapp et al., 1991	List of Massachusetts veterans who served between 1958 and 1973 and received a bonus	Vietnam service

continued

TABLE B-1 Continued

Reference	Design	Description	Sources of Exposure Data	Exposure Measures
American Legion Studies				
Snow et al., 1988	Cohort	Health and reproductive outcomes among American Legion members who served in Vietnam, examining combat and herbicide exposures	Questionnaire	Scale of combat intensity based on self-report
Stellman et al., 1988a	Cohort	Social and behavioral outcomes among American Legion members who served in Vietnam, examining combat and herbicide exposures	Questionnaire	Separate exposure opportunity indexes for Agent Orange and for all herbicides, based on 1986 proximity model using HERBS and Services HERBS tapes and point locations for centers of major troop activity
Stellman et al., 1988b	Cohort	Health and reproductive outcomes among American Legion members who served in Vietnam, examining combat and herbicide exposures	Questionnaire	Separate exposure opportunity indexes for Agent Orange and for all herbicides, based on 1986 proximity model using HERBS and Services HERBS tapes and point locations for centers of major troop activity

Other Studies of Vietnam Veterans

Aschengrau and Monson, 1989	Case-control	Paternal Vietnam service and risk of spontaneous abortion	Federal military records Massachusetts Vietnam bonus list	Vietnam service
Aschengrau and Monson, 1990	Case-control	Paternal Vietnam service and risk of late adverse pregnancy outcomes	Federal military records Massachusetts Vietnam bonus list	Vietnam service
Tarone et al., 1991	Case-control	Vietnam veterans with testicular cancer and hospital controls with other cancers	Questionnaire	Vietnam service

NOTES: Excludes studies of the Air Force Health Study (Ranch Hand) and Army Chemical Corps cohorts. CDC, Centers for Disease Control and Prevention; DMDC, Defense Manpower Data Center; EOI, exposure opportunity index; ESG, U.S. Army and Joint Services Environmental Support Group; NHL, non-Hodgkin's lymphoma; PTSD, posttraumatic stress disorder; STS, soft-tissue sarcoma; TCDD, 2,3,7,8-tetrachlorodibenzo-*p*-dioxin.
SOURCE: Adapted from Table C-3 (IOM, 2007).

REFERENCES

Anderson, H. A., L. P. Hanrahan, M. Jensen, D. Laurin, W. Y. Yick, and P. Wiegman. 1986. *Wisconsin Vietnam veteran mortality study: Final report.* Madison: Wisconsin Division of Health.

Aschengrau, A., and R. R. Monson. 1989. Paternal military service in Vietnam and risk of spontaneous abortion. *Journal of Occupational Medicine* 31(7):618–623.

Aschengrau, A., and R. R. Monson. 1990. Paternal military service in Vietnam and the risk of late adverse pregnancy outcomes. *American Journal of Public Health* 80(10):1218–1224.

Boehmer, T. K., W. D. Flanders, M. A. McGeehin, C. Boyle, and D. H. Barrett. 2004. Post-service mortality in Vietnam veterans: 30-year follow-up. *Archives of Internal Medicine* 164(17):1908–1916.

Boyle, C. A., P. Decouflé, R. J. Delaney, F. DeStefano, M. L. Flock, M. I. Hunter, M. R. Joesoef, J. M. Karon, M. L. Kirk, P. M. Layde, D. L. McGee, L. A. Moyer, D. A. Pollock, P. Rhodes, M. J. Scally, and R. M. Worth. 1987. *Postservice mortality among Vietnam veterans.* Atlanta, GA: Centers for Disease Control, U.S. Department of Health and Human Services.

Breslin, P., H. K. Kang, Y. Lee, V. Burt, and B. Shepard. 1988. Proportionate mortality study of US Army and US Marine Corps veterans of the Vietnam War. *Journal of Occupational Medicine* 30(5):412–419.

Bullman, T. A., H. K. Kang, and K. K. Watanabe. 1990. Proportionate mortality among U.S. Army Vietnam veterans who served in Military Region I. *American Journal of Epidemiology* 132(4):670–674.

Bullman, T. A., H. K. Kang, and T. L. Thomas. 1991. Posttraumatic stress disorder among Vietnam veterans on the Agent Orange Registry: A case-control analysis. *Annals of Epidemiology* 1(6):505–512.

Bullman, T. A, K. K. Watanabe, and H. K. Kang. 1994. Risk of testicular cancer associated with surrogate measures of Agent Orange exposure among Vietnam veterans on the Agent Orange Registry. *Annals of Epidemiology* 4:11–16.

Burt, V. L., P. P. Breslin, H. K. Kang, and Y. Lee. 1987. *Non-Hodgkin's lymphoma in Vietnam veterans.* Department of Medicine and Surgery, U.S. Veterans Administration, Washington, DC.

CDC (Centers for Disease Control and Prevention). 1987. Postservice mortality among Vietnam veterans. *Journal of the American Medical Association* 257(6):790–795.

CDC. 1988a. Health status of Vietnam veterans: I. Psychosocial characteristics. *Journal of the American Medical Association* 259(18):2701–2707.

CDC. 1988b. Health status of Vietnam veterans: II. Physical health. *Journal of the American Medical Association* 259(18):2708–2714.

CDC. 1988c. Health status of Vietnam veterans: III. Reproductive outcomes and child health. *Journal of the American Medical Association* 259(18):2715–2719.

CDC. 1988d. Serum 2,3,7,8-tetrachlorodibenzo-p-dioxin levels in U.S. Army Vietnam-era veterans. *Journal of the American Medical Association* 260(9):1249–1254.

CDC. 1989. *Health status of Vietnam veterans: Vietnam Experience Study.* Volumes I–V, Supplements A–C. Available: http://www.cdc.gov/nceh/veterans/default1c.htm (accessed December 21, 2007).

CDC. 1990a. The association of selected cancers with service in the U.S. military in Vietnam: I. Non-Hodgkin's lymphoma. *Archives of Internal Medicine* 150:2473–2483.

CDC. 1990b. The association of selected cancers with service in the U.S. military in Vietnam: II. Soft-tissue and other sarcomas. *Archives of Internal Medicine* 150:2485–2492.

CDC. 1990c. The association of selected cancers with service in the U.S. military in Vietnam: III. Hodgkin's disease, nasal cancer, nasopharyngeal cancer, and primary liver cancer. *Archives of Internal Medicine* 150:2495–2505.

CDC. 1990d. *The association of selected cancers with service in the U.S. military in Vietnam: Final report.* Atlanta, GA: U.S. Department of Health and Human Services.

Clapp, R. W. 1997. Update of cancer surveillance of veterans in Massachusetts, USA. *International Journal of Epidemiology* 26(3):679–681.

Clapp, R. W., L. A. Cupples, T. Colton, and D. M. Ozonoff. 1991. Cancer surveillance of veterans in Massachusetts, USA, 1982–1988. *International Journal of Epidemiology* 20(1):7–12.

Dalager, N. A., H. K. Kang, V. L. Burt, and L. Weatherbee. 1991. Non-Hodgkin's lymphoma among Vietnam veterans. *Journal of Occupational Medicine* 33(7):774–779.

Dalager, N. A., H. K. Kang, and T. L. Thomas. 1995a. Cancer mortality patterns among women who served in the military: The Vietnam experience. *Journal of Occupational and Environmental Medicine* 37(3):298–305.

Dalager, N. A., H. K. Kang, V. L. Burt, and L. Weatherbee. 1995b. Hodgkin's disease and Vietnam service. *Annals of Epidemiology* 5(5):400–406.

Decouflé, P., P. Holmgreen, C. Boyle, and N. Stroup. 1992. Self-reported health status of Vietnam veterans in relation to perceived exposure to herbicides and combat. *American Journal of Epidemiology* 135(3):312–323.

Deprez, R. D., M. E. Carvette, and M. S. Agger. 1991. *The health and medical status of Maine veterans: Final report.* Portland, ME: Public Health Resource Group, Inc.

Eisen, S., J. Goldberg, W. R. True, and W. G. Henderson. 1991. A co-twin control study of the effects of the Vietnam War on the self-reported physical health of veterans. *American Journal of Epidemiology* 134:49–58.

Erickson, J. D., J. Mulinare, P. W. McClain, T. G. Fitch, L. M. James, A. B. McClearn, and M. J. Adams, Jr. 1984a. *Vietnam veterans' risks for fathering babies with birth defects.* Atlanta, GA: U.S. Department of Health and Human Services, Centers for Disease Control and Prevention.

Erickson, J. D., J. Mulinare, P. W. McClain, T. G. Fitch, L. M. James, A. B. McClearn, and M. J. Adams, Jr. 1984b. Vietnam veterans' risks for fathering babies with birth defects. *Journal of the American Medical Association* 252(7):903–912.

Farberow, N. L., H. K. Kang, and T. A. Bullman. 1990. Combat experience and postservice psychosocial status as predictors of suicide in Vietnam veterans. *Journal of Nervous and Mental Disease* 178(1):32–37.

Fiedler, N., M. Gochfeld, and W. W. Lewis. 1992. *The Pointman Project: Neurobehavioral correlates of herbicide exposure in Vietnam veterans.* New Jersey Agent Orange Commission.

Goldberg, J., W. R. True, S. A. Eisen, and W. G. Henderson. 1990. A twin study of the effects of the Vietnam War on posttraumatic stress disorder. *Journal of the American Medical Association* 263(9):1227–1232.

Goun, B. D., and L. H. Kuller. 1986. *Final report: A case control study on the association of soft tissue sarcomas, non-Hodgkin's lymphomas, and other selected cancers and Vietnam military service in Pennsylvania males.* Pittsburgh, PA: University of Pittsburgh.

Greenwald, P., B. Kovasznay, D. N. Collins, and G. Therriault. 1984. Sarcomas of soft tissues after Vietnam service. *Journal of the National Cancer Institute* 73:1107–1109.

Holmes, A. P., C. Bailey, R. C. Baron, E. Bosanac, J. Brough, C. Conroy, and L. Haddy. 1986. *Vietnam-era veterans mortality study, West Virginia residents, 1968–1983: Preliminary report.* Charleston: West Virginia Department of Health.

IOM. 2007. *Veterans and Agent Orange: Update 2006.* Washington, DC: The National Academies Press.

Kahn, P. C., M. Gochfeld, M. Nygren, M. Hansson, C. Rappe, H. Velez, T. Ghent-Guenther, and W. P. Wilson. 1988. Dioxins and dibenzofurans in blood and adipose tissue of Agent Orange-exposed Vietnam veterans and matched controls. *Journal of the American Medical Association* 259(11):1661–1667.

Kahn, P. C., M. Gochfeld, and W. W. Lewis. 1992a. *Immune status and herbicide exposure in the New Jersey Pointman I Project.* New Jersey Agent Orange Commission.

Kahn, P. C., M. Gochfeld, and W. W. Lewis. 1992b. *Semen analysis in Vietnam veterans with respect to presumed herbicide exposure.* Pointman II Project. New Jersey Agent Orange Commission.

Kang, H. K., L. Weatherbee, P. Breslin, Y. Lee, and B. Shepard. 1986. Soft tissue sarcomas and military service in Vietnam: A case comparison group analysis of hospital patients. *Journal of Occupational and Environmental Medicine* 28(12):1215–1218.

Kang, H. K., F. Enziger, P. Breslin, M. Feil, Y. Lee, and B. Shepard. 1987. Soft tissue sarcoma and military service in Vietnam: A case-control study. *Journal of the National Cancer Institute* 79(4):693–699.

Kang, H. K., C. M. Mahan, K. Y. Lee, C. A. Magee, S. H. Mather, and G. M. Matanoski. 2000a. Pregnancy outcomes among U.S. women Vietnam veterans. *American Journal of Industrial Medicine* 38:447–454.

Kang, H. K., C. M. Mahan, K. Y. Lee, C. A. Magee, and S. Selvin. 2000b. Prevalence of gynecologic cancers among female Vietnam veterans. *Journal of Occupational and Environmental Medicine* 42(11):1121–1127.

Kogan, M. A., and R. Clapp. 1985. *Mortality among Vietnam veterans in Massachusetts, 1972–1983.* Office of the Commissioner of Veterans' Services, Agent Orange Program. The Commonwealth of Massachusetts.

Kogan, M. A., and R. Clapp. 1988. Soft tissue sarcoma mortality among Vietnam veterans in Massachusetts, 1972–1983. *International Journal of Epidemiology* 7(1):39–43.

Lawrence, C. E., A. A. Reilly, P. Quickenton, P. Greenwald, W. F. Page, and A. J. Kuntz. 1985. Mortality patterns of New York State Vietnam veterans. *American Journal of Public Health* 75:277–279.

Levy, C. J. 1988. Agent Orange exposure and posttraumatic stress disorder. *Journal of Nervous and Mental Disease* 176(4):242–245.

Mahan, C. M., T. A. Bullman, and H. K. Kang. 1997. A case-control study of lung cancer among Vietnam veterans. *Journal of Occupational and Environmental Medicine* 39(8):740–747.

McKinney, W. P., D. D. McIntire, T. J. Carmody, and A. Joseph. 1997. Comparing the smoking behavior of veterans and nonveterans. *Public Health Reports* 112:212–217.

Newell, G. R. 1984. Development and preliminary results of pilot clinical studies: Report of the chairman. Agent Orange Advisory Committee to the Texas Department of Health.

O'Brien, T. R., P. Decouflé, and C. A. Boyle. 1991. Non-Hodgkin's lymphoma in a cohort of Vietnam veterans. *American Journal of Public Health* 81(6):758–760.

Pollei, S., F. A. Mettler, Jr., C. A. Kelsey, M. R. Walters, and R. E. White. 1986. Follow-up chest radiographs in Vietnam veterans: Are they useful? *Radiology* 161:101–102.

Rellahan, W. 1985. *Aspects of the health of Hawaii's Vietnam-era veterans reflecting the impact of the Vietnam experience.* Hawaii Department of Health.

Snow, B. R., J. M. Stellman, S. D. Stellman, and J. F. Sommer, Jr. 1988. Post-traumatic stress disorder among American Legionnaires in relation to combat experience in Vietnam: Associated and contributing factors. *Environmental Research* 47(2):175–192.

Stellman, J. M., S. D. Stellman, and J. F. Sommer, Jr. 1988a. Social and behavioral consequences of the Vietnam experience among American Legionnaires. *Environmental Research* 47(2):129–149.

Stellman, J. M., S. D. Stellman, and J. F. Sommer, Jr. 1988b. Utilization, attitudes, and experiences of Vietnam era veterans with Veterans Administration health facilities: The American Legion experience. *Environmental Research* 47(2):150–174.

Tarone, R. E., H. M. Hayes, R. N. Hoover, J. F. Rosenthal, L. M. Brown, L. M. Pottern, N. Javadpour, K. J. O'Connell, R. E. Stutzman. 1991. Service in Vietnam and risk of testicular cancer. *Journal of the National Cancer Institute* 83(20):1497–1499.

Thomas, T. L., H. K. Kang, and N. A. Dalager. 1991. Mortality among women Vietnam veterans, 1973–1987. *American Journal of Epidemiology* 134(9):973–980.

True, W. R., J. Goldberg, and S. A. Eisen. 1988. Stress symptomatology among Vietnam veterans. *American Journal of Epidemiology* 128(1):85–92.

Visintainer, P., M. Barone, H. McGee, and E. L. Peterson. 1995. Proportionate mortality study of Vietnam-era veterans of Michigan. *Journal of Occupational and Environmental Medicine* 37(4):423–428.

Watanabe, K. K., and H. K. Kang. 1995. Military service in Vietnam and the risk of death from trauma and selected cancers. *Annals of Epidemiology* 5:407–412.

Watanabe, K. K., and H. K. Kang. 1996. Mortality patterns among Vietnam veterans. *Journal of Occupational and Environmental Medicine* 38(3):272–278.

Watanabe, K. K., H. K. Kang, and T. L. Thomas. 1991. Mortality among Vietnam veterans: With methodological considerations. *Journal of Occupational and Environmental Medicine* 33(7):780–785.

Wendt, A. S. 1985. *Iowa Agent Orange survey of Vietnam veterans*. Iowa State Department of Health.

Appendix C

Biographical Sketches of Committee Members

David A. Savitz, Ph.D. (*Chair*), is the Charles W. Bluhdorn Professor of Community and Preventive Medicine and director of the Epidemiology, Biostatistics, and Disease Prevention Institute at the Mount Sinai School of Medicine. Dr. Savitz's primary research activities and interests are in reproductive, environmental, and cancer epidemiology. His teaching is focused on epidemiologic methods, and he authored a book entitled *Interpreting Epidemiologic Evidence*. He is past president of the Society for Epidemiologic Research and of the Society for Pediatric and Perinatal Epidemiologic Research. He has served on several Institute of Medicine and National Research Council studies, including the Committee on EPA's Exposure and Human Health Reassessment of TCDD and Related Compounds and the Committee on Understanding Premature Birth and Assuring Healthy Outcomes. He served as vice chair of the Committee on the Possible Effects of Electromagnetic Fields on Biologic Systems. He has authored over 200 peer-reviewed journal articles and is currently an editor of *Epidemiology*. He was elected a member of the Institute of Medicine in 2007.

Mehran Alaee, Ph.D., is a research scientist at Environment Canada, with a research focus on the sources and fate of persistent organic pollutants in the environment. He served as principal investigator for a study of the impact of polybrominated diphenyl ethers on the Canadian environment and the health of Canadians. He is a member of the International Advisory Board for Dioxin Symposia as well as the International Advisory Board for Brominated Flame Retardants workshops. He was co-chair for Dioxin 2005, the 25th International Symposium on Halogenated Environmental

Organic Pollutants and Persistent Organic Pollutants, as well as for BFR 2004, the 3rd International Symposium on Brominated Flame Retardants in the Environment. He coordinates the Environmental Interest Group of the American Society for Mass Spectrometry and serves on the editorial board for *Chemosphere* (Persistent Organic Pollutants and Dioxins section). Dr. Alaee received his Ph.D. in analytical chemistry from the University of Guelph, Ontario.

Francesca Dominici, Ph.D., is a professor in the Department of Biostatistics of the Bloomberg School of Public Health at the Johns Hopkins University. Dr. Dominici has extensive experience in the development of statistical methods and their applications to clinical trials, toxicology, biology, and environmental epidemiology. Dr. Dominici has led the development of statistical and epidemiological methods for analyzing a national database on air pollution, weather, and mortality. She is a member of the American Statistical Association and the International Biometric Society. Dr. Dominici is the recipient of the first Walter A. Rosenblith Young Investigator Award from The Health Effects Institute of Boston, the 2001 Young Investigator Award of the American Statistical Association, and the 2006 Mortimer Spiegelman Award from the American Public Health Association. She earned her Ph.D. in statistics from the University of Padua, Italy. Dr. Dominici has served the National Academies as a member of the Committee on Gulf War and Health: Review of the Medical Literature Relative to Gulf War Veterans' Health and the Committee to Assess Potential Health Effects from Exposures to PAVE PAWS Low-level Phased-array Radiofrequency Energy.

Gurumurthy Ramachandran, Ph.D., is a professor in the Division of Environmental Health Sciences at the University of Minnesota's School of Public Health. His research interests include occupational and ambient exposure assessment, Bayesian methods in retrospective exposure assessment, exposure modeling, mathematical methods for analyzing occupational measurements, occupational hygiene decision making, and inhalation dosimetry for mixed exposures. Dr. Ramachandran has written extensively on occupational environmental assessment, including a textbook on occupational exposure assessment. He is a Certified Industrial Hygienist. He earned his bachelor's degree in electrical engineering from the Indian Institute of Technology, Bombay; his M.S. in environmental engineering from the Virginia Polytechnic Institute and State University; and his Ph.D. in environmental sciences and engineering from the University of North Carolina at Chapel Hill.

William G. Seibert, M.A., is the senior archivist and chief of the Archival Operations Branch at the National Archives and Records Administration's

National Personnel Records Center (NPRC) in St. Louis. He has worked with NARA's collections of twentieth-century military personnel and medical records for nearly 30 years and has wide knowledge of alternate record sources available for use in reconstructing military service and medical data. In July 2004 he was appointed chief of the Archival Operations and Facility Planning Branch of the Center's newly established Archival Programs Division. As the Center's preservation officer from 2000 to 2004, he was responsible for establishing NPRC's archival preservation program, building and equipping its preservation laboratories, and recruiting its 24-person staff of preservation specialists and technicians. Prior to 2000 he headed the Military Organizational Records Appraisal and Disposition Project at the Center. The purpose of this project, begun in 1976, is to identify and archive permanently valuable material contained in the Center's 100,000-cubic-foot collection of mid-twentieth-century program and administrative records of Army, Air Force, and Navy field commands. Mr. Seibert served for two and one half-years in the U.S. Army. He received his A.B. in history from the College of William and Mary and his B.A. and M.A. in law from the University of Oxford. He was a charter member of the Academy of Certified Archivists and is affiliated with the Society of American Archivists and the Association of St. Louis Area Archivists.

Leslie T. Stayner, Ph.D., is professor and director of the Division of Epidemiology and Biostatistics at the University of Illinois at Chicago School of Public Health. Before joining the university in 2003, Dr. Stayner was chief of the Risk Evaluation Branch, Education and Information Division, of the National Institute for Occupational Safety and Health. He also served as visiting scientist at the International Agency for Research in Cancer in Lyon, France, in 2001–2002. His research interests include occupational, environmental, and chronic disease epidemiology, epidemiologic methods, and risk assessment. Dr. Stayner is a fellow of the American College of Epidemiology and the Institute of Medicine of Chicago, and he is a member of the Society for Epidemiologic Research, the American Public Health Association, and the International Commission on Occupational Health. He received his M.Sc. in Epidemiology and Occupational Health and Safety from the Harvard School of Public Health and his Ph.D. in epidemiology with a formal minor in biostatistics from the University of North Carolina. Dr. Stayner previously served on the National Research Council Committee on Human Health Risks of Trichloroethylene.

Lance A. Waller, Ph.D., is a professor in the Department of Biostatistics at Emory University. Dr. Waller's research interests involve statistical analysis of spatial patterns in public health data. Past investigations include development of statistical tests of spatial clustering in disease incidence data and implementation of spatial and space–time Markov random field models for maps of disease rates. He is currently investigating statistical methods to analyze environmental exposure, demographic, and disease incidence data linked through geographic information systems (GISs). His ongoing research projects involve assessment of environmental justice, local measures of health disparities, and the distribution of epidermal nerve fibers in the skin. Dr. Waller earned his Ph.D. in operations research from Cornell University. He has served the National Academies as a member of the Committee to Assess Potential Health Effects from Exposures to PAVE PAWS Low-level Phased-array Radiofrequency Energy and the Committee on Review of Existing and Potential Standoff Explosives Detection Techniques.

Mary H. Ward, Ph.D., is an investigator in the Occupational and Environmental Epidemiology Branch in the Division of Cancer Epidemiology and Genetics at the National Cancer Institute. Her research interests include cancer risks associated with environmental exposure to pesticides and other chemicals; and the role that N-nitroso compounds and their precursors play in cancer development, particularly exposure to nitrate from drinking water and diet. Cancers of specific interest include childhood leukemia, non-Hodgkin's lymphoma, colorectal, and stomach cancer. Dr. Ward has incorporated state-of-the art exposure assessment into her studies by developing interdisciplinary collaborations with environmental scientists, environmental engineers, hydrogeologists, geographers, and biostatisticians to estimate exposure to environmental contaminants based on environmental monitoring data, land use maps, and geographic fate and transport models. She received an M.S. in ecology from the University of Tennessee and a Ph.D. in epidemiology from the Johns Hopkins School of Hygiene and Public Health. Dr. Ward serves as an associate editor for *Environmental Health Perspectives* and on the EPA Board of Scientific Counselor's Drinking Water Subcommittee, which reviews EPA's drinking water research program.

Thomas F. Webster, D.Sc., is an associate professor in the Department of Environmental Health at the Boston University School of Public Health and deputy director and a principal investigator of the Boston University Superfund Basic Research Program. His research interests include methods in environmental epidemiology (particularly spatial epidemiology and ecologic bias) and application of mathematical modeling to toxicology and epidemiology. A second major research interest involves the sources, fate, and hazards of dioxins and other persistent organic compounds. A current project investigates exposure routes and body burdens of polybrominated diphenyl ethers. Dr. Webster served on the organizing committee for Dioxin

2003, the 23rd International Symposium on Halogenated Environmental Organic Pollutants and Persistent Organic Pollutants, and on the NRC Committee on Fluoride in Drinking Water.

Susan R. Woskie, Ph.D., is professor in the Department of Work Environment, School of Health and Environment, at the University of Massachusetts at Lowell. Her research interests include exposure assessment for occupational epidemiologic studies, biomarkers of exposure, toxicokinetic modeling, and developing methods to integrate total exposure assessment into epidemiology and risk assessment. Dr. Woskie serves on the editorial board of the *American Journal of Occupational and Environmental Hygiene* and on the advisory panel for the Agricultural Health Study, which is sponsored by the National Cancer Institute, the National Institute of Environmental Health Sciences, and the Environmental Protection Agency. She was a member of the Institute of Medicine Committee to Review the Health Effects in Vietnam Veterans of Exposure to Agent Orange and Herbicides (Second Biennial Update) and the Committee to Review the Evidence Regarding the Link between Exposure to Agent Orange and Diabetes. She received her M.Sc. in environmental health/industrial hygiene at the Harvard School of Public Health and her Ph.D. in biomedical science/industrial hygiene from Clark University.